Blood Gases in
Clinical Practice

Blood Gases in Clinical Practice

By

LEOPOLDO LAPUERTA, M.D.
Chairman, Department of Medicine
Medical Director of Respiratory Therapy
Santa Rosa Medical Center
Clinical Assistant Professor
Department of Medicine
University of Texas Medical School
San Antonio, Texas

With a Foreword by

Sydney Schiffer, M.D.
Clinical Professor
Department of Medicine
University of Texas
Health Science Center
San Antonio, Texas

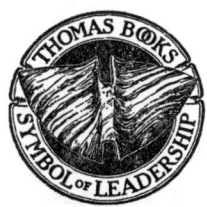

CHARLES C THOMAS · PUBLISHER
Springfield · Illinois · U.S.A.

Published and Distributed Throughout the World by
CHARLES C THOMAS • PUBLISHER
BANNERSTONE HOUSE
301-327 East Lawrence Avenue, Springfield, Illinois, U.S.A.

This book is protected by copyright. No part of it
may be reproduced in any manner without written
permission from the publisher.

© *1976, by* CHARLES C THOMAS • PUBLISHER
ISBN 0-398-03527-X
Library of Congress Catalog Card Number: 75-34298

With THOMAS BOOKS *careful attention is given to all details of manufacturing and design. It is the Publisher's desire to present books that are satisfactory as to their physical qualities and artistic possibilities and appropriate for their particular use.* THOMAS BOOKS *will be true to those laws of quality that assure a good name and good will.*

Printed in the United States of America
N-1

Library of Congress Cataloging in Publication Data

Lapuerta, Leopoldo.
   Blood gases in clinical practice.

   Bibliography: p.
   Includes index.
   1. Inhalation therapy. 2. Blood gases. I. Title. [DNLM: 1. Blood gas analysis. 2. Intensive care units. 3. Critical care. QY450 L317b]
RM161.L36   615' .836   75-34298
ISBN 0-398-03527-X

FOREWORD

Dr. Lapuerta's book on blood gases is based on a many-year experience in San Antonio's leading hospitals, as physician in charge of pulmonary services, and as a bed-side clinician and teacher. His approach, therefore, is simple and basic and meant to be of use to practicing physicians, nurses and inhalation therapy technicians. As such, the book will receive widespread distribution and usage as did his previous *Manual of Respiratory Failure*, published in 1972 and an immediate success for the same reasons —a minimum of theory and a maximum of practical application.

Sydney Schiffer, M.D.

INTRODUCTION

THE HUMAN BODY HAS a delicate balance of physical chemical factors which is necessary for life to be sustained. Metabolic processes are taking place continuously in different organs. Oxygen is being used. Chemical reactions occur with the intervention of enzymes. CO_2 is being produced. Other waste products are formed and need to be removed. The basic organs of intake are the lungs (oxygen) and the gastrointestinal system (food stuffs and water). The cardiovascular system is the basic mechanism of transportation. The two most important organs for the output are the lungs (CO_2) and the kidneys (water, electrolytes and waste products). The central nervous system is instrumental in maintaining respiration, controlling many vital functions and, often forgotten but also vitally important, maintaining the proper relationship with the environment necessary for survival (eating when hungry, closing the glottis to prevent aspiration, reacting to pain, etc.)

In order for the heart to continue pumping the blood and for many enzymatic reactions to take place, it is necessary that some physical and chemical conditions remain stable within a relatively narrow margin. The pressure of the cardiovascular system must stay between given values. The temperature cannot deviate excessively from the normal. Concentration of some chemicals of the blood, such as hydrogen ions, potassium, glucose, etc., has to remain within a given range. The fluids of the body have to have in solution an amount of oxygen adequate to supply the metabolic needs of the tissues.

Life is interrupted when the internal mileu is such that it cannot support brain metabolism or myocardial contraction. When in an agonic patient the heart rate slows, the QRS wave of the electrocardiogram widens and the contractions of the cardiac muscle finally cease, more often than not, the immediate cause for this stoppage of the heart is an excessive concentration of hydrogen ions in the blood (acidemia) or a lack of adequate oxygen supply to the myocardium. When in another patient the heart suddenly goes into ventricular fibrillation, we know that its irritability is greatly increased, perhaps because there are excessive concentrations of foreign substances (i.e., Digitalis®) in the blood, or because some other compounds (potassium, calcium) are present in abnormal proportions. All of this can occur in hearts which are basically normal.

Failure of the lungs to perform their function for a few minutes (drowning, respiratory arrest) or failure of the other intake (gastrointestinal system) and output (kidneys) organs for days or weeks will create internal conditions incompatible with life unless necessary corrective action is taken.

When practicing intensive care medicine, we have to deal with all the above considerations and problems. And some of these problems present themselves in critically ill patients regardless of whether the initial abnormality was pneumonia, myocardial infarction, diarrhea or any other clinical entity. Etiological treatment of disease is indeed very important and not to be neglected. But intensive medicine concerns itself very intimately with supportive therapy of vital functions and with the maintenance of an internal milieu in which these vital functions can take place.

Therapy could be considered at three different levels:

1. *Mechanical,* such as bypassing an intestinal obstruction, removing a tumor, ventilating an apneic patient;

2. *Pharmacological,* giving a drug to alter the functions of the body or of its infecting organisms;

3. *Supportive or replacement therapy,* such as removing excessive amounts of waste products by hemodialysis, administering water and electrolytes to replace excessive losses, etc.

Ancient medical practices have given birth to modern pharmacological medicine. Engineering concepts and ancient surgery have evolved into our present surgical techniques. Supportive and replacement therapy, however, have been possible only after reliable instruments have been developed to measure physical phenomena and chemical substances. The development of the blood pressure cuff, intravascular pressure measuring devices, chemical methods of determining concentrations of electrolytes and other substances in the blood, the pH and blood gases electrodes, all have brought significant advancements in our understanding of the critically ill patient and have given us the tools with which we can fight and on occasions conquer disease.

Intensive medicine is, to a great extent, quantitative medicine. Things are measured and, if significantly abnormal, corrected. Technology and precision are very important. We cannot ventilate mechanically a patient in respiratory failure without adequate measurements of blood gases and ventilatory volumes any more than we can treat diabetic acidosis by squirting insulin in the veins without precise dosages and blood sugar controls. Since therapeutic decisions are made many times in the light of laboratory results, good training, experience and a sense of responsibility in the medical and paramedical personnel is essential in intensive medicine. Lack of objectivity is as dangerous as ignorance. In intensive medicine, guessing is wrong when measuring is possible; yet, on the other hand, we need a keen sense of clinical observation and an ability to differentiate the important from the marginal, along with a basic knowledge of physiopathology, not to be misled by a barrage of data that may not always be accurate.

It is the intent of the author to put together some basic facts, thoughts, and therapeutic approaches that hopefully will assist the reader to use the determinations of blood gases and pH for the welfare of the patients. This book is not intended to be a textbook on intensive medicine. Rather, it contains some basic material that the author, through several years of experience in intensive care units, has found to be what residents, interns, intensive care unit nurses and respiratory care technicians need most to understand. Some concepts are so basic that their explanation may appear offensive at first glance to the obviously trained intensive care worker. But experience tells us that basic concepts are not always really understood by everyone who makes decisions in the care of a critically ill patient.

I do not want to give the impression that determination of

blood gases is the answer for every critical situation. They are a test, and like any other test they are no better than the mind that would make judicious use of it. How much to use them and how aggressive to be in therapy as a result of the knowledge that they provide depends mainly on our personal effort to improve our knowledge and our objectivity. Aggressiveness or conservatism in treating a patient should not be part of our mental framework. We should always do what is best for the patient, which at times may require just holding back without taking any action and at times may call for many therapeutic maneuvers. I hope that this book may be of some help to the reader in following this path of objectivity.

CONTENTS

	Page
Foreword	v
Introduction	vii

Chapter
- I. REVIEW OF SOME PHYSICAL CHEMICAL FACTS 3
  - Movement of Gases: Mass Movement and Diffusion ... 3
  - Solution of Gases in Water 5
  - Transport of Gases in Blood 7
  - Acidity of the Blood 10
- II. PHYSIOLOGICAL CONSIDERATIONS ABOUT BLOOD GASES AND ACID-BASE BALANCE 14
  - General Considerations 14
  - Pulmonary Physiology 15
  - Elimination of CO_2 16
  - Oxygenation 17
  - Technique of Obtaining Arterial Blood for Gas Analysis 20
  - General Guidelines in the Interpretation of Arterial Blood Gases 22
  - Changes in the pCO_2 28
  - Changes in Plasma Bicarbonate 29
  - Oxygenation 32
  - Relationship Between Blood Gases and Electrolytes ... 34
- III. SYMPTOMS DUE TO ABNORMALITIES OF THE BLOOD GASES .. 38
  - Hypercapnea 38
  - Acidemia 38
  - Hypoxia 39
  - Hypocapnea 40
  - Alkalemia 40
  - Hyperoxygenation 41

Chapter	Page
Combined Abnormalities	42
IV. GENERAL GUIDELINES OF THERAPY IN PROBLEMS OF OXYGENATION, VENTILATION AND ACID-BASE BALANCE	43
Problems of Oxygenation	43
Problems of Acid-Base Balance and Ventilation	45
V. BLOOD GASES IN CHRONIC OBSTRUCTIVE LUNG DISEASE	50
General Considerations	50
Treatment of Chronic Obstructive Lung Disease	53
Treatment of the Compensated Phase of Chronic Lung Disease	54
Treatment of the Decompensated Phase of Chronic Lung Disease	59
VI. MECHANICAL VENTILATION	64
Choice of Ventilator	64
Ventilation	65
Oxygenation	68
Humidification and Temperature Control	69
Practical Points in the Care of the Patient During Mechanical Ventilation	69
The Process of Weaning the Patient from Mechanical Ventilation	74
VII. BLOOD GASES IN ACUTE PULMONARY EDEMA	76
VIII. BLOOD GASES IN CARDIAC ARREST	82
IX. BLOOD GASES IN NEUROLOGICAL DISORDERS	89
Cerebrovascular Accident	89
Psychogenic Hyperventilation	91
Epileptic Attack	93
Arteriosclerosis of the Cerebrovascular System	94
Overdose	95
X. BLOOD GASES IN NEUROMUSCULAR DISORDERS	97
The Guillain-Barre Syndrome	97
Poliomyelitis	98
Myasthenia Gravis	98
Amyotrophic Lateral Sclerosis	100

Chapter	Page
Tetanus	100
XI. BLOOD GASES IN THE RESPIRATORY DISTRESS SYNDROME OF THE ADULT	101
XII. BLOOD GASES IN MISCELLANEOUS PROBLEMS	107
Chest Wall Problems	107
Drowning and Near Drowning	109
Index	111

Blood Gases in
Clinical Practice

CHAPTER I

REVIEW OF SOME PHYSICAL CHEMICAL FACTS

MOVEMENT OF GASES: MASS MOVEMENT AND DIFFUSION

A GAS OR A MIXTURE of gases moves rapidly from an area of higher to one of lower total pressure provided that there is no mechanical barrier in between. This is why an inflated rubber balloon, with its inside air at higher than atmospheric pressure, deflates rapidly when the neck is left open. This is also why the air rushes in and out of the lungs with the respiratory excursions. We know that when the wind blows from the North, barometric pressure North of town is higher than South. All of these are examples of *mass movement* of gases. In such a movement, all molecules of gas move together, regardless of their nature. A mixture of gases behaves no different in this respect than a pure gas does. The driving force here is the difference in total gas pressure and the movement is usually rapid.

By contrast, *diffusion* of a gas is based upon a different principle. When moving by diffusion, the molecules of a gas go from a higher to a lower partial pressure of such a gas, independently of the total pressure of the mixture of gases and also independently of the nature of the other gases. As we open a bottle of perfume in the corner of a room, the scent will be noticed in the opposite corner within a given time, even if the air in the room is quiet. In diffusion, molecules of a gas are able to go through permeable membranes and are also able to change phase, this is, going from a liquid to gas phase or vice versa. The three basic characteristics that differentiate diffusion of gases from mass movement are then:

1. The driving force in diffusion is the difference in partial pressure of the gas in question, not the total gas pressure.

2. In their diffusion, gas molecules can go through membranes.
3. In their diffusion, gas molecules can change phase.

The following experiment demonstrates the two first characteristics (Fig. 1). A rubber balloon is filled with air and the neck securely tied. The balloon is then introduced in a larger box that has an inlet and an outlet and one of the walls is transparent for observation. With both inlet and outlet open, CO_2 gas is introduced from a tank into the box through the inlet while gases are allowed to exit through the outlet. After a few minutes of appropriate gas flow, we have practically washed out the air of the box and replaced it by CO_2. The inlet is closed first and in a few seconds the outlet is also closed. In such a situation, total gas pressure inside a box is the same as atmospheric, but practically only CO_2 gas is producing it. Inside the balloon, pressure is higher than atmospheric and the gases responsible for it are mainly

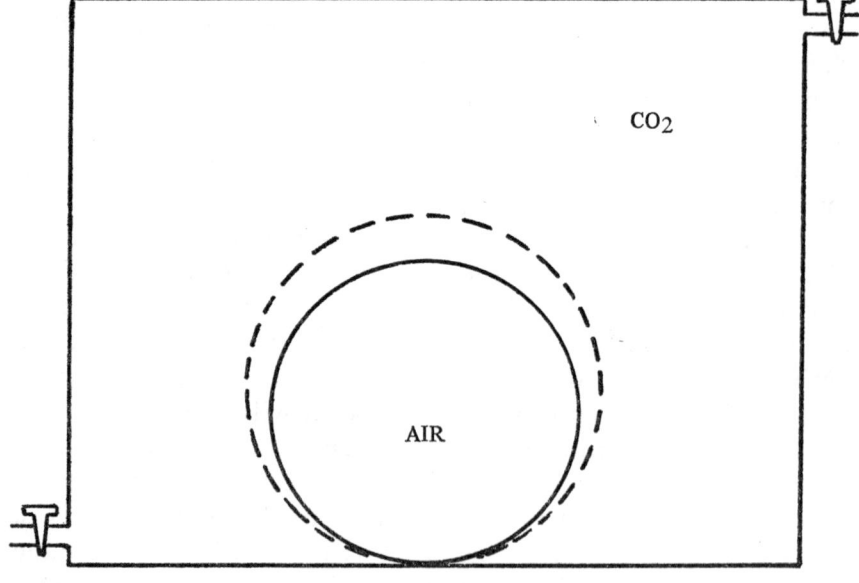

Figure 1. Diffusion of gases. A rubber balloon filled with air and placed in CO_2 at atmospheric pressure keeps expanding until bursting, because the CO_2 diffuses into the balloon, through the rubber wall, faster than O_2 and N_2 diffuse out.

nitrogen and oxygen. In the next several hours, the balloon keeps getting bigger and bigger inside the box until it finally bursts. The CO_2 diffuses through a rubber membrane faster than oxygen and nitrogen do. Since the initial partial pressure of CO_2 in the box is atmospheric and inside the balloon close to zero, CO_2 gas diffuses rapidly from the outside to the inside. On the other hand, nitrogen and oxygen diffuse from the inside to the outside but they do it at a much slower rate. As a result, the total volume inside the balloon keeps increasing until it bursts. The CO_2 has diffused into the balloon clearly against a higher total pressure and through a membrane.

A simple example of a gas changing phase in its diffusion would be the loss of the crispy taste of soda water when the bottle is left open. The CO_2 dissolved in the water diffuses to the air and its concentration in water decreases.

Air moves in and out of the lungs by the mechanical action of mass movement but exchange of gases between alveolar air and blood occurs by diffusion.

SOLUTION OF GASES IN WATER

Gases can dissolve in water as well as solids do. We can dissolve oxygen, CO_2 and nitrogen in water as easily as we dissolve salt or sugar. Dissolved gases can even change the taste of the water. Compare the taste of tap water (usually with oxygen and nitrogen dissolved) with that of soda water (high amounts of CO_2 dissolved) and that of recently boiled water (practically no gas dissolved). Dissolved gas can be extracted from the water and measured. The quantity of a given gas dissolved in a sample of water depends on the nature of the gas, the temperature of the water and the partial pressure of the gas in the mixture of gases with which the water is in contact. The warmer the water, the less gas can be held in solution. The higher the partial pressure of the gas, the more of it is held in solution. As an example, if we have water at 37° Centigrade in contact with pure oxygen at a pressure of 760 mm Hg, once equilibrium between water and gas is reached, each cc of water will contain 0.02365 cc's of oxygen. In the case of CO_2, in similar circumstances, the figure would be

0.518. These numbers represent the *solubility coefficient* of oxygen and CO_2 respectively in water at 37° Centigrade. The solubility of CO_2 in water is approximately twenty-five times greater than that of oxygen.

As indicated before, gases change phase by diffusion. We also have said that gases always diffuse from the higher to the lower partial pressure. It is then obvious that when equilibrium between a mixture of gases and a liquid has been reached in a way that a particular gas is not moving from one phase to the other, the partial pressure of such a gas in the two phases is the same. In the example described in the previous paragraph, we know that when oxygen at 760 mm Hg of pressure is in equilibrium with water the partial pressure of oxygen dissolved in the water is also 760 mm, Hg. Therefore, *the partial pressure of a gas dissolved in a liquid is the same partial pressure that this gas has in the mixture of gases with which the liquid stands in equilibrium.* As we apply this to the physiology of gas exchange, it would mean that the partial pressure of oxygen, CO_2 and nitrogen in the alveolar air is the same as that in the capillary blood that is returning to the left atrium, since most of the time complete equilibrium between gases of the alveolar air and the capillary blood is achieved.

TABLE I

SYMBOLS USED TO EXPRESS THE PARTIAL PRESSURES OF OXYGEN, CO_2 AND NITROGEN

Symbol	Partial Pressure of
PIO_2	Oxygen in inspired air
$PICO_2$	CO_2 in inspired air
PIN_2	Nitrogen in inspired air
PAO_2	Oxygen in alveolar air
$PACO_2$	CO_2 in alveolar air
PAN_2	Nitrogen in alveolar air
$p\bar{c}O_2$	Oxygen in capillary blood
$p\bar{c}CO_2$	CO_2 in capillary blood
$p\bar{c}N_2$	Nitrogen in capillary blood
paO_2	Oxygen in Arterial blood
$paCO_2$	CO_2 in arterial blood
paN_2	Nitrogen in arterial blood
$p\bar{v}O_2$	Oxygen in mixed venous blood
$p\bar{v}CO_2$	CO_2 in mixed venous blood
$p\bar{v}N_2$	Nitrogen in mixed venous blood

Table I shows the different symbols used to express the partial pressures of the three basic gases in the inspired air, in the alveoli, in the capillary blood, in the arterial blood and in the mixed venous blood.

TRANSPORT OF GASES IN BLOOD

As far as solution of gases is concerned, blood behaves basically like water. The concepts of pO_2 and pCO_2 discussed above apply to blood in the same manner. But if the transport of gas in blood were to take place by solution alone, impractically large amounts of blood would be needed. From the solubility coefficients of oxygen and CO_2 on water at 37° Centigrade given above, we can calculate that even at a partial pressure of 760 mm Hg, only 23.65 cc of oxygen could be held in solution in a liter of blood. At a normal paO_2 of 90 mm Hg, the amount of oxygen dissolved in one liter of blood would be only 2.8 cc. For each mm Hg of paO_2 a liter of blood would have $\frac{23.65}{760} = 0.031$ cc of O_2, and 100 cc of blood would have 0.0031 cc of O_2. In contrast, at a partial pressure of 760 mm Hg, a liter of blood could contain in solution 518 cc's of CO_2. This would be approximately $\frac{518}{760} = 0.68$ cc of CO_2 per mm Hg of pCO_2, and at a normal arterial pCO_2 of 40 mm Hg the amount of CO_2 dissolved in one liter of blood would be 27.2 cc (2.72 cc of CO_2 per 100 cc of blood).

It is obvious that while transport of CO_2 could theoretically be accommodated in a water-like circulatory liquid, the transport of oxygen could not. This obstacle to oxygen transport is solved by the presence of the hemoglobin in the red cells. Hemoglobin stores oxygen, and also some CO_2, in chemical combination. The amount of oxygen stored in the hemoglobin of a sample of blood depends mainly on the magnitude of the pO_2 in that blood and also, understandably, on the amount of hemoglobin available.

When fully saturated, one gram of hemoglobin will hold approximately 1.38 cc of oxygen (the oxygen being measured at standard conditions of temperature, pressure and dryness). The degree of saturation of hemoglobin with oxygen in relationship to the pO_2 of the blood is expressed in the oxygen-hemoglobin-dissociation curve. The curve is affected, among other things, by the temperature of the blood, its degree of acidity (pH) and its pCO_2. A standard dissociation curve of 37° Centigrade, pH of 7.4 and pCO_2 of 40 mm Hg is presented in figure 2.

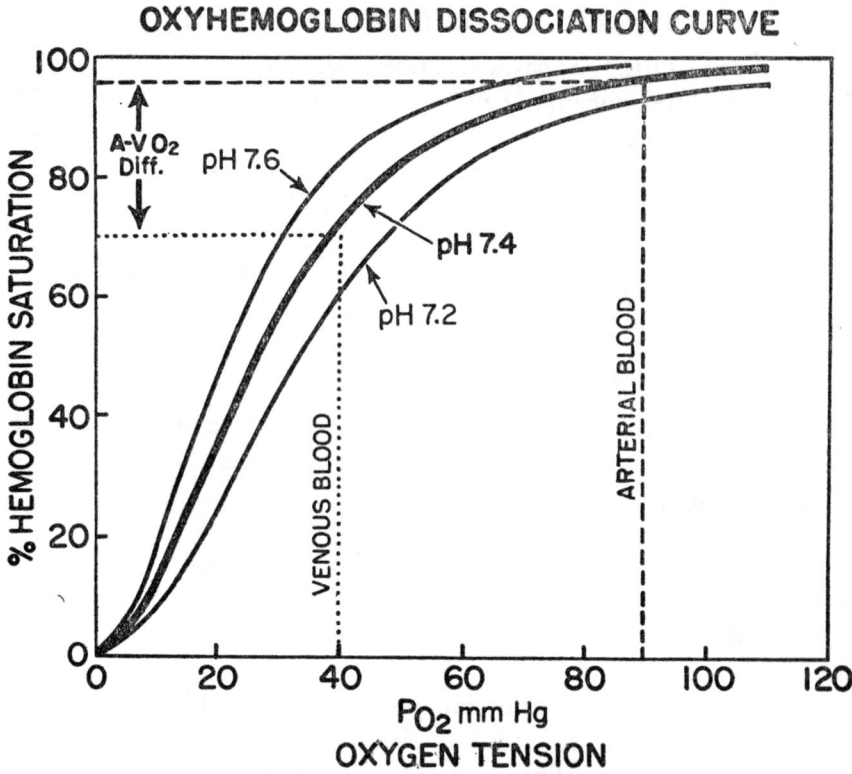

Figure 2. Oxygen-Hemoglobin dissociation curve at 37° C. and pCO_2 at 40 mm Hg. From Andrews, Joseph L., *Clinical Notes on Respiratory Diseases.* 13:2, 9, 1974. Reproduced with the permission of the American Lung Association.

Many other factors can affect the affinity of hemoglobin for oxygen, such as the amount of carbon monoxide present, the quality of the hemoglobin itself, the presence of other chemicals or enzymes in the blood, etc. Carbon monoxide is perhaps the most important of these factors, not only in the cases of acute carbon monoxide intoxication, but also in many other situations.

A heavy smoker that consumes two to three packages of cigarettes a day may have as much as 20 percent or more of his hemoglobin combined with carbon monoxide, leaving only the rest for the transport of oxygen. In experimental conditions, a 20-pound dog will die of tissue hypoxia due to carbon monoxide intoxication after inhaling the smoke of five or six cigarettes in a period of one hour when the burning cigarette is incorporated into the circuit of a mechanical ventilation device that sustains the ventilation of the dog.

The following concepts are of importance when studying oxygen transport:

Oxygen capacity of a sample of blood is the amount of oxygen which is contained in the hemoglobin of 100 cc of such blood when the hemoglobin is fully saturated with oxygen. In an approximate manner, it could be calculated by multiplying the hemoglobin in grams percent by 1.38.

Oxygen saturation of a sample of blood is the relationship between the amount of oxygen that is contained in its hemoglobin and the amount that would be contained if the hemoglobin were fully saturated with oxygen.

Oxygen content of a sample blood is the real amount of oxygen in cc's contained in 100 cc's of such blood. It comprises the oxygen combined with the hemoglobin and the oxygen dissolved. From what has been said so far, the oxygen content can be calculated as follows:

$$\text{Oxygen content (in cc)} = \frac{\% \; O_2 \text{ saturation} \cdot O_2 \text{ capacity}}{100} + pO_2 \cdot 0.0031$$

Examples: With the standard dissociation curve, and with a hemoglobin of 15 grams percent and a pO_2 of 90 mm Hg, the following approximate values will be obtained:

O_2 capacity $= 15 \cdot 1.38 = 20.7$ in cc's per 100 cc of blood

O_2 saturation $= 96.87\%$

O_2 content $= \frac{96.87 \cdot 20.7}{100} + 90 \cdot 0.0031 = 20.05 + 0.28 = 20.33$ in cc's per 100 cc of blood.

The hemoglobin plays a much less essential role in the transport of carbon dioxide because of the much greater solubility of this gas in water. Furthermore, the hemoglobin-CO_2 dissociation curve is relatively close to a straight line (Fig. 3). Since in cases of anemia or hemoglobin poisoning, the transport of oxygen is affected to a critical level much sooner than the transport of CO_2 can be seriously disturbed, we will consider that for practical purposes in most cases of clinical medicine there is no significant problem with the transport of CO_2, provided that circulation is maintained.

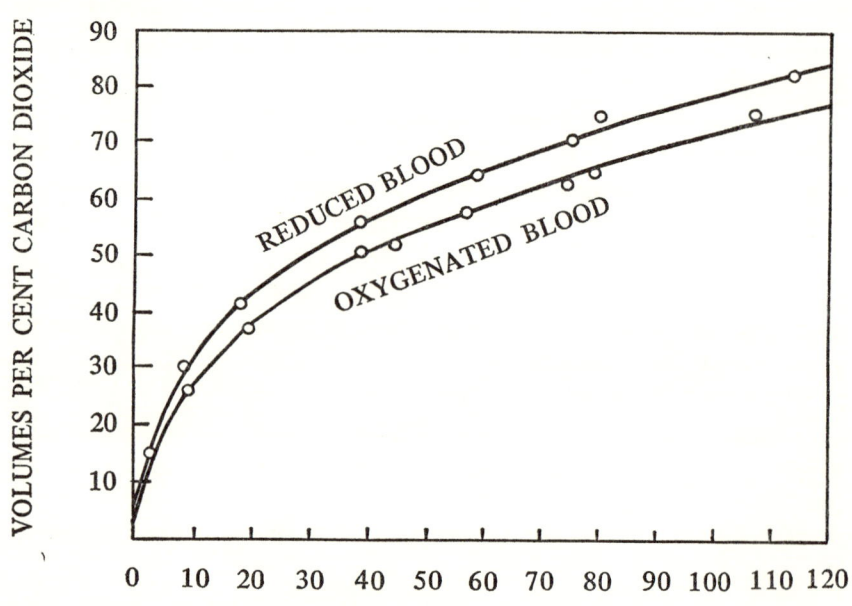

Figure 3. Hemoglobin-CO_2 dissociation curve.
From data of Christiansen, et. al.: "The Adsorption and Dissociation of Carbon Dioxide by Human Blood." *J. Physiol.* (London), *48*:244, 1914.

Table II shows the approximate normal values of many of the measurements, previously discussed, in arterial and mixed venous blood.

ACIDITY OF THE BLOOD

Whenever there is water, there are some Hydrogen ions (H^+) in solution, because some H_2O molecules dissociate into OH^-

Review of Some Physical Chemical Facts

TABLE II
NORMAL VALUES OF DIFFERENT GAS MEASUREMENTS IN ARTERIAL AND IN MIXED VENOUS BLOOD, WHEN THE HEMOGLOBIN IS 15 AND THE Hb-O_2 DISSOCIATION CURVE IS STANDARD

	Arterial Blood	
	O_2 Capacity	20.7 cc per 100 cc of blood
	paO_2	90 mm Hg (85-100)
	O_2 Saturation	96.87% (96.5 to 97)
	O_2 Content	20.33 cc per 100 cc of blood (20 to 20.5)
	$paCO_2$	40 mm Hg (35 to 45)
	Mixed Venous Blood	
	O_2 Capacity	Same as in arterial blood
	$p\bar{v}O_2$	40 mm Hg (35 to 45)
	O_2 Saturation	74% (72-76)
	O_2 Content	15.14 cc per 100 cc of blood (14 to 16)
	$p\bar{v}CO_2$	46 mm Hg (41 to 51)

and H^+. Pure water has approximately one gram of Hydrogen ions per ten million liters. Therefore, one liter of pure water has 0.0000001 grams of Hydrogen ions.

Since one Mol of H^+ weighs approximately one gram, it follows that:

one liter of H_2O has 0.0000001 mol H^+, or

0.0001 millimols (mM), or 0.1 nannomols.

Also, one liter of H_2O has 0.0000001 grams H^+, or $\frac{1}{10,000,000}$ grams or

10^{-7} grams.

Since pH of a solution is defined as the negative of the decimal logarithm of the concentration of H^+ in grams per liter, it follows that the pH of pure water is the negative of -7, this is, 7.

An acid is a solution with more H^+ than water. A base is a solution with less H^+ than water. Therefore, an acid is a solution with a concentration of H^+ greater than 0.0001 mg/liter, or a pH lower than 7. Similarly, a base is a solution with a concentration of H^+ lower than 0.0001 mg/liter, or with a pH higher than 7.

An acid, when added to pure water, increases the H^+ concentration of the water. A base when added to pure water, decreases the H+ concentration of the water.

In the blood, the concentration of H+ ([H+]) is regulated by a buffer system where the main base is sodium bicarbonate ($NaHCO_3$) and the main acid is carbonic acid (H_2CO_3). With some simplification, it can be said that $[H^+] \cong \frac{[H_2CO_3]}{[NaHCO_3]}$. With the sign $\cong$ meaning "Proportional to."

Since $pH \cong \frac{1}{[H^+]}$, it can be said that $pH \cong \frac{[NaHCO_3]}{[H_2CO_3]}$

The exact relationship between pH, bicarbonate and carbonic acid is expressed by the Henderson-Hasselbalch equation:

$$pH = pk' + \log_{10} \frac{\text{bicarbonate in mEq/L}}{H_2CO_3 \text{ in mM/L}}$$

Since H_2CO_3 is the product of the combination of CO_2 and H_2O, we could substitute CO_2 in mM/L for H_2CO_3 in mM/L. Knowing the solubility coefficient of CO_2 and the factor needed to transform cc's of CO_2 gas in mM/L at 37°, it can be said that CO_2 in mM/L = $pCO_2 \cdot 0.03$. The Henderson-Hasselbalch equation can then be written as follows:

$$pH = pk' + \log_{10} \frac{\text{bicarbonate in mEq/L}}{pCO_2 \text{ in mm Hg} \cdot 0.03}$$

Since the pk' of the buffer system of the blood is very close to 6.1, the normal bicarbonate concentration is 24 mEq/L and the normal arterial pCO_2 is 40 mm Hg, in a sample of normal blood the pH can be calculated as follows:

$$pH = 6.1 + \log_{10} \frac{24}{40 \cdot 0.03} = 6.1 + \log_{10} \frac{24}{1.2} = 6.1 + \log_{10} 20 = 6.1 + 1.3 = 7.4.$$

It can be seen that normal blood has a little higher pH than pure water. But for practical reasons, we will accept 7.4 as the neutral point of the blood. That is, blood with a pH above 7.43 will be called alkaline and with a pH below 7.37 will be accepted as acidic.

The use of pH as a measurement of the concentration of H+ in the blood seems to be a little confusing since it is based on the determination of the negative of a logarithmic figure and, as such, it changes in opposite direction than the concentration of H+. A more logical approach would appear to be the use of concentration of H^+ by itself. But in this book we will continue to use the concept of pH because of its wider acceptance at the present time.

REFERENCES

Bartels, H. et al.: *Methods in Pulmonary Physiology.* New York: Hafner, 1963.

Comroe, J.: *Physiology of Respiration,* 2nd ed. Chicago: Year Bk Med, 1966.

Comroe, J. et al.: *The Lung: Clinical Physiology and Pulmonary Function Tests.* Chicago: Year Bk Med, 1962.

Fenn, W. O., and Rahn, H.: *Handbook of Physiology,* Section 3, *Respiration.* Baltimore: Williams and Wilkins, 1964.

Filley, G. F.: *Acid-base and Blood Gas Regulation.* Philadelphia: Lea and Febiger, 1972.

CHAPTER II

PHYSIOLOGICAL CONSIDERATIONS ABOUT BLOOD GASES AND ACID-BASE BALANCE

GENERAL CONSIDERATIONS

IN DEALING WITH THE critically ill patient, one of the most important tasks is to maintain an internal milieu in which the vital organs can function properly. Total blood volume, effectiveness of cardiac output, state of contraction of peripheral vessels, hydrostatic pressure of the blood in arteries, veins and heart chambers are very important factors. Physicians and nurses working in Intensive Medicine should have the knowledge of the physiology, monitoring and therapy related to these factors. In this book, however, we are concerning ourselves specifically with the composition of the blood itself as a basic condition for the proper sustainment of vital functions. We will particularly focus our discussions on how to maintain in the blood the proper amounts of H^+, Oxygen, CO_2 and some of the basic electrolytes.

Maintaining the pH within proper limits is critical for the survival of the patient. The heart of a healthy adult would most likely cease to beat effectively when the pH falls below 6.8. In ill individuals with abnormalities of myocardial function, oxygenation, electrolyte balance, etc., a drop of the pH to 7.0 or 7.1 may be fatal. The tolerance to higher than normal pH is less well established. Young, healthy individuals have been seen to briefly increase their pH to 7.9 by voluntary hyperventilation without serious damage. But by clinical experience, we know that a seriously ill patient will most likely develop serious complications when the pH is 7.6 or more for prolonged periods of time.

High and low pCO_2 can have significant effect in the overall condition of the patient by their influence on the pH, but also by the specific changes they may produce in the cerebral vasculature and by their effect on the respiratory center.

Changes in the concentration of plasma bicarbonate by themselves may not produce any symptoms, but they are certainly of the utmost importance because of their influence on the pH of the blood. Too high or too low a concentration of oxygen in the blood may also have significant pathophysiological consequences. Death is preceded in most instances by a period of time during which oxygen, CO_2 and H^+ concentrations in the blood are progressively deteriorating. Understanding of their changes and of the possible therapeutic maneuvers to reverse them may be critical for the survival of the patient.

We will analyze initially the blood gases as a product of the function of the lungs and this will be followed by a discussion of the general guidelines for interpretation of blood gas abnormalities. The relationship of the blood gases to blood electrolytes will be discussed and we will try to elaborate on some general therapeutic considerations. The clinical usefulness of blood gases in specific diseases or clinical situations will be discussed later.

PULMONARY PHYSIOLOGY

We will be referring to *ventilation* as the process by which air or a different mixture of gases is moved in and out of the lungs. This is a mechanical process which requires proper function of central nervous system, peripheral nerves and respiratory muscles, as well as patent airways and healthy lung tissue. Adequate ventilation is essential for the proper removal of carbon dioxide from the blood.

Oxygenation, on the other hand, is the process by which adequate supplies of oxygen are being introduced into the blood stream. Some degree of ventilation of course is necessary in the process of oxygenation, because oxygen has to reach the alveoli before it can be transferred to the blood. But in considering oxygenation, other factors become vitally important, such as the structural integrity of the lungs and the concentrations of oxygen used.

By *acid-base balance,* we understand the relationship between concentration of H+ in the blood, plasma bicarbonate and dissolved CO_2 gas. The function of the lungs is essential here because of the importance of the concentration of CO_2 gas, but a second factor equally important will be the concentration of plasma bicarbonate.

ELIMINATION OF CO_2

CO_2 is being produced in the tissues at a rate of approximately 200-250 cc per minute at rest. Production during exercise may increase to as much as ten times that amount. The CO_2 produced in the tissues diffuses freely toward the blood and is carried by circulation to the lungs. In the lung tissue, it diffuses from capillary blood to alveolar air and is finally carried out of the lungs by the mechanical act of ventilation. Since there is no clinical condition that would significantly impair diffusion of CO_2 from capillary blood to alveolar air when circulation is maintained effectively, *the only possible cause of CO_2 retention would be inadequacy of ventilation.*

An average-size adult person would breathe, at rest, approximately ten to sixteen times per minute (respiratory rate) and would move in each breath in and out of the lungs approximately 500 cc of air (tidal volume). The total amount of air moved in and out in a minute will be between 5 and 8 liters (minute ventilation).

Respiratory rate $\times$ tidal volume $=$ minute ventilation

Of the 500 cc of air that enter the respiratory system in one breath, only approximately three-fourths will reach an area of the lungs into which CO_2 gas is diffusing. The remaining fourth of the tidal volume stays in the airways and doesn't receive any CO_2. This space where some inspired air remains without receiving CO_2 is called *physiological dead space.* During expiration, the air of the physiological dead space comes out first, practically unchanged in its composition, except for the fact that water vapor has saturated it. Air that has received CO_2 in the lungs and has given oxygen to the blood will follow. This is called *alveolar air.*

When the dead space air and the alveolar air exhaled are

measured not only in a single breath but in all the breaths taken in one minute, we can calculate the *dead space ventilation* and *alveolar ventilation*.

The important thing in maintaining adequate levels of arterial pCO_2 is to have an alveolar ventilation commensurate with the CO_2 production. A panting respiration, even if it has a very high minute ventilation on account of a very rapid rate, may not lower the pCO_2 of the blood because very little air in each breath reaches the alveoli. On the contrary, with very deep breaths and a slow rate, we may accomplish increased alveolar ventilation without increasing the minute ventilation. Physiological dead space is not a fixed number for each patient. It changes also according to the depth of the breath, since increased stretching of the lungs dilates more the airways. Figure 4 shows the relationship between tidal volume and physiological dead space in a series of our patients.

When the CO_2 production and the physiological dead space are both very much increased, we may need a very high minute ventilation with high tidal volume to maintain adequate arterial pCO_2. This is the case of some of the patients with the acute respiratory distress syndrome of the adult in which, at times, we have had to use tidal volumes of 1000 cc with minute ventilations of as much as 25 liters. Increased minute ventilation during exercise in healthy individuals is primarily intended to match the increased CO_2 production.

Particular problems of ventilation will be discussed later in the book as we review hypercapnia and the different disease entities.

OXYGENATION

In order to maintain adequate levels of oxygen in the blood, not only must we have an efficient ventilation that would provide exchange of gases between alveoli and the outside, but it is also necessary to have the right conditions in the lung itself that would allow for sufficient transfer of oxygen from the alveolar air to the blood. In contrast to ventilation, the *composition* of the gas used in breathing is very important in the process of oxygenation.

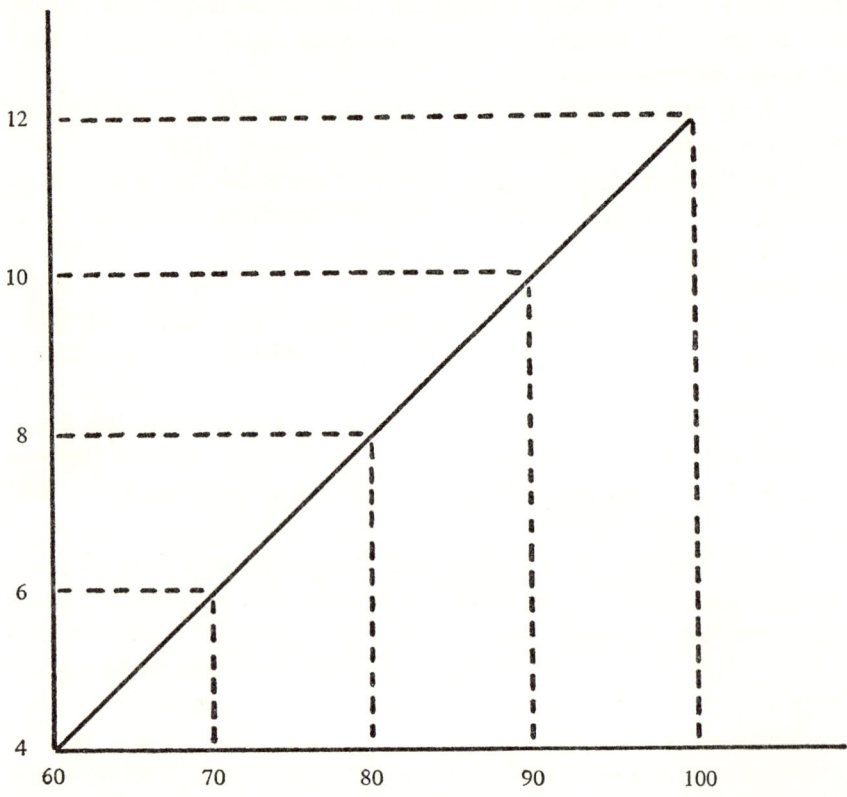

Figure 4. Relationship between physiological dead space and tidal volume.

Physiological dead space is expressed as percentage of the content of air in the lung at that time during inspiration, this is, functional residual capacity plus the particular tidal volume used.

The numbers in the abscissa represent the above mentioned measurement (functional residual capacity plus tidal volume) as percentage of the total lung capacity.

Once a reasonably effective ventilation is achieved, the single most important factor in determining what the level of oxygen in the blood would be in a particular patient is the concentration of oxygen in the inspired air. A patient may be ventilating sufficiently and still be hypoxic when breathing room air if there is damage to the structure in the lungs. Yet, the same patient may ventilate much less but use a higher percentage of oxygen in the inspired air and would have perhaps very good oxygen content, even if he is retaining CO_2.

TABLE III
CAUSES OF LOW ARTERIAL pO_2

1. Low concentration of O_2 in inspired air (low F_IO_2)
2. Hypoventilation with normal F_IO_2
3. Abnormality of the lung tissue:
    a. Right to left shunt
    b. Abnormal ventilation perfusion relationship
    c. Diffusion defect

The possible causes of arterial hypoxemia (low arterial pO_2) are shown in Table III. Low concentration of oxygen in the inspired air (Low F_IO_2), even if very important in physiological studies of respiration at high altitude, is not a problem in the daily clinical practice of the average hospital. Decreased ventilation is, of course, of primary importance in case of cardiorespiratory arrest and in drowning. It also plays a significant role in the hypoxemia of advanced cases of pulmonary edema and of advanced cases of respiratory failure. But in most chronically or subacutely ill respiratory patients, the main cause of hypoxemia resides in the abnormal structure of the diseased lung. Right to left shunt is seen in cases of pneumonia, pulmonary infarction, respiratory distress syndrome of the adult and of the newborn, congenital cardiopathies, and a variety of other clinical situations. Abnormal ventilation perfusion relationship is the most common cause of hypoxemia in chronic obstructive disease of the lungs and in acute asthmatic attacks. Diffusion defect is a phenomenon that very seldom occurs as a main cause of hypoxemia. After an extensive study of the problem, we have data to support the idea that it occurs in some extreme cases of hypoxemia, but indeed is not a very frequent phenomenon that we encounter in clinical practice.

Regardless of the physiopathological explanation for the hypoxia, we can in most instances increase the arterial pO_2 by increasing the concentration of inspired oxygen. How to do this or indeed whether or not to do it at all is a matter of judgement that would differ from one clinical situation to another and this will be discussed later in the book as we review different disease entities.

On the other hand, lowering of an abnormally high pCO_2 is always accomplished by increasing alveolar ventilation, regardless of the composition of the gas being used.

TECHNIQUE OF OBTAINING ARTERIAL BLOOD FOR GAS ANALYSIS

The technique of obtaining blood for gas analysis is simple and safe. We use a #25 needle for infants and small children and a #23 for older children and adults. In newborns or very small infants, repeated arterial punctures may not be feasible and in such cases we may have to cannulize the umbilical artery or to use arterialized capillary blood. But when arterial blood is obtainable, capillary or venous blood should not be used. We use a 2 cc or 5 cc glass syringe. If the hub of the needle is transparent, obtention of the blood is easier. The first drop of blood is seen immediately as it reaches the hub, indicating that the lumen of the artery has been reached, making perforation of the posterior wall or repeated puncture of the artery less likely. The syringe and needle are first prepared with a small amount of 1 to 1,000 Heparin solution, just enough to fill the dead space of these instruments (too much Heparin will alter the pH of the withdrawn blood). We do not use a local anesthetic in adult patients in order to avoid possible drug reactions and because the pain of the arterial puncture is usually no greater than the pain that would accompany the injection of the anesthetic.

We prefer to use the radial artery. It has the advantage of being superficial. When the wrist is slightly extended the radial artery is usually relatively well fixed between the skin and the harder deep layers of muscle and bone. If a hematoma forms after a puncture it is more easily identified in the area of the radial than it would be in the brachial or femoral artery. If the artery were to be seriously injured, the collateral circulation from the ulnar artery will give sufficient perfusion to the hand in most cases. Even if our preference is the radial artery, the brachial and femoral can also be used, and with good technique, the puncture is safe.

In general, we obtain 1 or 2 ml of blood, depending on the type of blood gas analyzer available. Once the first drop of blood comes spontaneously into the hub of the needle, the syringe will start filling by itself. However, once we are satisfied that we are obtaining arterial blood, a gentle suction may hasten withdrawal. After removal of the needle, pressure should be applied to the site of the puncture for three or four minutes. The operator may be fully satisfied at the time of discontinuing pressure that no further bleeding is occurring. The responsibility of containing possible hemorrhage should not be delegated to untrained assistants.

It should be emphasized that when properly done, the arterial puncture is a safe procedure. In many scores of thousands of these punctures, we have not had a single significant complication. Every interested physician should be able to perform an arterial puncture properly. Nurses and well-trained respiratory care technicians should be allowed to perform these punctures when a physician is not available, since the benefits to be obtained from the immediate use of such determinations are enormous and far exceed the risk of complications.

Once the blood is withdrawn, a gentle rotation of the syringe will insure proper mixing of Heparin and blood. In large and very active intensive care units, it is recommended that the blood gas machine be kept standardized at all times in the unit. If the determination of pH and blood gases is to be done immediately, no cooling of the blood is necessary. When more than two or three minutes will elapse between drawing and determination, the blood should be stored in ice.

There are several pH and blood gas analyzers on the market. If the hospital is to make efficient use of blood gas determinations, it is important that the blood gas and pH meter be standardized twenty-four hours a day and ready for use at any time. Emergency situations, such as cardiac arrest, serious metabolic acidosis and acute respiratory failure may need prompt action which will be guided by the values obtained in blood gas determinations. The direct measurements obtained from the blood gas analyzer are the pH, pO_2 and pCO_2. From these determinations, easy calculation can give in a matter of seconds the value for oxygen hemoglobin saturation and the plasma bicarbonate.

GENERAL GUIDELINES IN THE INTERPRETATION OF ARTERIAL BLOOD GASES

A set of blood gases usually comprises the values of the pH, pCO_2, plasma bicarbonate, pO_2 and oxygen saturation of the hemoglobin. In some instances, the value of the base excess is added. In interpreting the blood gases, we have found it helpful to mentally separate the problem of oxygenation from that of the ventilation and acid-base balance. We will be studying them separately.

Ventilation and acid-base balance. The interpretation of ventilation and acid-base balance problems concerns independently and collectively three figures: The pH, the pCO_2 and the plasma bicarbonate of the blood.

pH is usually the most important determination. A pH between 7.37 and 7.43 is usually accepted as normal. A pH below 7.36 represents acidemia which could be described as mild (between 7.36 and 7.30), moderate (between 7.29 and 7.25) or severe (below 7.24). pH below 6.8 is usually incompatible with life. A pH above 7.43 represents alkalemia which we will consider as mild (between 7.44 and 7.50), moderate (between 7.51 and 7.6) or severe (above 7.6).

pCO_2. We usually consider as normal a pCO_2 between 35 and 45 mm Hg. pCO_2's above 45 mm Hg represent hypercapnea. Values below 35 mm Hg indicate the existence of hypocapnea. Hypercapnea is always the result of insufficient alveolar ventilation. Hypocapnea is always due to increased alveolar ventilation.

Plasma bicarbonate. Plasma bicarbonate levels between 23 and 25 mEq per liter are usually considered normal. Hyperbasemia exists when the plasma bicarbonate is 26 mEq per liter or more. Concentrations of 22 mEq per liter or less constitute hypobasemia. The terms "mild," "moderate" and "severe" hyper or hypobasemias are not particularly appropriate because the

Physiological Considerations About Blood Gases

severity of a clinical situation will depend on the value of pH rather than on the value of the plasma bicarbonate by itself.

pCO_2 and plasma bicarbonate are the two basic factors that will determine the value of the pH. As indicated in Chapter I, the Henderson-Hasselbalch equation shows how the interaction of plasma bicarbonate and pCO_2 will produce the pH:

$$pH = pk' + \log_{10} \frac{\text{Plasma Bicarbonate in mEq/L}}{pCO_2 \text{ in mm Hg} \cdot 0.03}$$

In clinical practice, a simplified form of the Henderson-Hasselbalch equation will help in understanding the nature and significance of the abnormalities encountered:

$$pH \cong \frac{\text{Bicarbonate}}{pCO_2}$$

Where the sign $\cong$ means "approximately equal to." It is seen in the equation that the pH can be lowered by either decreasing the plasma bicarbonate or by an increase of the pCO_2. On the contrary, the pH will be increased by an increase of the bicarbonate or by a decrease of the pCO_2. If the bicarbonate and pCO_2 both increase or decrease in the same proportion, the pH will remain unchanged.

Changes in the concentration of the plasma bicarbonate correspond to what the classic literature in acid-base balance has been calling "metabolic abnormalities." Changes in the values of the pCO_2 have been classically called "respiratory abnormalities." In some countries there is a tendency to talk about "chemical" changes when the bicarbonate is involved and "gaseous" changes when the pCO_2 is involved. No matter what terminology we use, we always come back to the same basic facts: The concentration of plasma bicarbonate and the level of pCO_2 may change and by so doing they may change the pH. It should be emphasized that the pH is the *result* of the interaction of the bicarbonate and the pCO_2 and that in order to change the pH we will have to alter the concentration of plasma bicarbonate or the pCO_2.

Four basic abnormalities of the acid-base balance have been described over the years. They are most commonly referred to in the English literature as metabolic acidosis, respiratory acidosis, metabolic alkalosis and respiratory alkalosis. The terms acidosis and alkalosis are somewhat vague in their meaning but are mostly accepted as indicating excessive amounts of total body acids or excessive amounts of total body base respectively. We think that it is more useful clinically not to focus primarily in such considerations of total acid or base in the body but rather on what the value of the pH or the concentration of hydrogen ions is in the blood as a result of the interaction of the acids and the bases of the body. For this reason, we think that the terms acidemia and alkalemia are more appropriate because they seem to indicate whether the blood has more or less hydrogen ions than normal. We will be then talking about metabolic acidemia, metabolic alkalemia, respiratory acidemia and respiratory alkalemia.

We could also approach the problem of the acidity of the blood by expressing it in terms of the concentration of hydrogen ions rather than pH. Some pulmonary and renal physiologists prefer to do so. We think that the idea is certainly logical. It would eliminate the exponential factors involved in the calculation of the pH. It would also eliminate the confusion of using lower numbers to express higher acidity and vice versa.

However, since the use of pH is so widely accepted, we will follow tradition in this respect and will continue to use the concept of the pH in this book instead of that of concentration of hydrogen ions.

Definition of the aforementioned abnormalities with examples of blood gases will follow:

Respiratory acidemia. Respiratory acidemia is the clinical condition in which the pH of the patient is low as a result of having a high pCO_2. A high pCO_2 is always due to poor alveolar ventilation.

Example: pH 7.1, pCO_2 80 mm Hg, bicarbonate 24 mEq per liter, or

$$\downarrow\downarrow \text{pH} \cong \frac{\text{Bicarbonate} \rightarrow}{pCO_2 \uparrow\uparrow}$$

Metabolic acidemia. Metabolic acidemia is a condition in which the pH of the blood is low as a result of having a low bicarbonate.

Example: pH 7.1, pCO_2 40 mm Hg, bicarbonate 12 mEq per liter, or

$$\downarrow\downarrow pH \cong \frac{\text{Bicarbonate} \downarrow\downarrow}{pCO_2 \rightarrow}$$

Respiratory alkalemia. Respiratory alkalemia is the condition in which the pH of the blood is high as a result of having a low pCO_2. Low pCO_2 is always a result of increased alveolar ventilation.

Example: pH 7.6, pCO_2 25 mm Hg, bicarbonate 24 mEq per liter, or

$$\uparrow\uparrow pH \cong \frac{\text{Bicarbonate} \rightarrow}{pCO_2 \downarrow\downarrow}$$

Metabolic alkalemia: Metabolic alkalemia is a condition in which the pH of the blood is high as a result of having a high concentration of plasma bicarbonate.

Example: pH 7.6, pCO_2 40 mm Hg, bicarbonate 40 mEq per liter, or

$$\uparrow\uparrow pH \cong \frac{\text{Bicarbonate} \uparrow\uparrow}{pCO_2 \rightarrow}$$

In the above examples, and throughout the book, we use the system of the abbreviated Henderson-Hasselbalch equation and we use arrows pointing up or down to indicate the deviation of the values from the normal. A horizontal arrow would mean normal value. We have found this system particularly good for didactic purposes. By expressing graphically the direction in which the bicarbonate and the pCO_2 are changing, their effect on the pH is clearly shown. Changes of the same proportion on the bicarbonate and the pCO_2 will cancel each other as far as the effect of pH is concerned. As an example, if a patient has double bicarbonate (48 mEq per liter) and double pCO_2 (80 mm Hg) than normal, the pH will remain at a normal of 7.4:

$$\rightarrow pH \cong \frac{\text{Bicarbonate} \uparrow\uparrow}{pCO_2 \uparrow\uparrow}$$

When the proportion of change of one of the two measurements is greater than the other, even if both go in this same direction, the pH will be altered by the component that changes the most.

Example: ph 7.25, pCO₂ 28, bicarbonate 12.

$$\downarrow pH \cong \frac{\text{Bicarbonate} \downarrow\downarrow}{pCO_2 \downarrow}$$

In this case the bicarbonate is half the normal and the pCO₂ has decreased by only 30 percent. As a result, the decrease in the bicarbonate is what determines the direction of change of the pH, in this case toward the acidic side.

If the two components change in opposite directions, as an example the pCO₂ increasing and the bicarbonate decreasing, the effect on the pH will be cumulative and a marked abnormality of the pH can be expected.

Example: pH 7.0, pCO₂ 64, bicarbonate 15 mEq per liter, or

$$\downarrow\downarrow\downarrow pH \cong \frac{\text{Bicarbonate} \downarrow\downarrow}{pCO_2 \uparrow}$$

A second example, this time bringing the pH to the alkaline side, would be a combination of high bicarbonate and low pCO₂, as follows:

pH 7.60, pCO₂ 31, bicarbonate 27.8, or

$$\uparrow\uparrow pH \cong \frac{\text{Bicarbonate} \uparrow}{pCO_2 \downarrow}$$

These combinations of abnormalities of the plasma bicarbonate and the pCO₂ are the rule rather than the exception in clinical practice. The four basic abnormalities described before very rarely present themselves in the isolated manner in which we have shown them for didactical purposes. A typical example of partial compensation of one abnormality by the other, often encountered in clinical practice, is the case of the "metabolic acidemia" of the young decompensated diabetic. On occasions, the accumulation of acids in the blood of the diabetic is such that it decreases the concentration of plasma bicarbonate to as little as 1 mEq per liter or less. This would produce a drop in pH so great that life would no longer be possible but, fortunately, most diabetics in that position will be stimulated to hyperventilate as a result of having a low pH, and by so doing they will reduce the arterial pCO_2 sufficiently as to partially compensate the drop of the pH and maintain it within a range compatible with life. A typical example would be as follows:

pH 7.0, pCO_2 17 mm Hg, bicarbonate 3 mEq per liter, or

$$\downarrow\downarrow\downarrow pH \cong \frac{\text{Bicarbonate} \downarrow\downarrow\downarrow\downarrow}{pCO_2 \downarrow\downarrow}$$

A typical example of the abnormalities of plasma bicarbonate and pCO_2 combining to produce a very serious drop in the pH is found in terminal stages of some patients with acute pulmonary edema. The pulmonary edema itself acts as an impairment to ventilation and in very difficult situations the pCO_2 increases, lowering the pH (respiratory component). But when the situation is very desperate, the low pH, along with the severe hypoxia generated by the pulmonary edema itself, reduces the transport of oxygen to the peripheral tissues so much that anaerobic metabolism takes place and great amounts of lactic acid is produced, which in turn destroys part of the bicarbonate and further decreases the pH (metabolic component). Example:

$$\downarrow\downarrow\downarrow pH \cong \frac{\text{Bicarbonate} \downarrow}{pCO_2 \uparrow\uparrow}$$

Because practically all combinations of abnormalities in the pCO_2 and the plasma bicarbonate are possible, a great variety of acid-base abnormalities are encountered in clinical practice. Since certain types of abnormalities have been encountered associated frequently in clinical practice with given disease identities, there has been a tendency to create labels with clinical connotations to designate such abnormalities of the acid-base balance. The reader will undoubtedly hear, on occasions, such terms as "compensated respiratory acidosis, hypochloremic alkalosis, etc." Rather than using such terms, we think that it is easier to obtain a clear picture of the abnormality of the acid-base balance by analyzing the three basic figures first independently and then drawing a composite picture. As an example, if we are faced with the following set of values:

pH 7.60, pCO_2 42 mm Hg, plasma bicarbonate 42 mEq per liter, the analysis of the situation would be as follows:

The pH is high (alkalemia). The plasma bicarbonate is high (hyperbasemia). The pCO_2 is maintained within normal limits. Therefore, the increase in pH is due to an increase in the plasma bicarbonate. The written interpretation that we would give to this set of values would be: "A high concentration of plasma bicarbonate is producing a high pH (metabolic alkalemia). Alveolar ventilation still remains within normal limits."

CHANGES IN THE pCO_2

The value of the arterial pCO_2 depends exclusively on the adequacy of alveolar ventilation to remove the CO_2 which has poured into the blood from the tissues. When the pCO_2 of the blood is high, it is so because the alveolar ventilation is not sufficient, regardless of whether or not the patient is in respiratory distress. Conversely, a low pCO_2 is always due to alveolar hyperventilation. Hyper and hypoventilation refer to the amount of air that moves in and out of the lungs and not to the rate of breathing. We still see nurses coming out of school having learned that hyperventilation consists of breathing fast. This is a wrong concept and such a deficiency in the use of terms should be corrected. Some patients with rapid breathing may be hyperventilating, but others may actually hypoventilate if the depth of their breaths is not adequate. A typical example can be seen in a panting dog. The tidal volume of the panting is so small that most of it stays in the physiological dead space and only a very minimal amount of air enters the alveolar spaces. As a result, the respiratory rate and the minute ventilation are quite high but alveolar ventilation is not increased and the arterial pCO_2 remains normal. In some cases of acute respiratory failure the patient may maintain a very rapid and shallow breathing, clearly insufficient to remove the CO_2 being produced, even at respiratory rates as high as forty or fifty per minute.

The most common causes of hypoventilation encountered in

clinical practice are: Chronic obstructive lung disease, severe cerebrovascular accident, pharmacological depression of the respiratory center, various neuropathies, severe trauma to the chest, etc.

Hyperventilation occurs frequently in cases of advanced cerebral arteriosclerosis, some intracranial lesions, psychogenic hyperventilation, excessive aggressive mechanical ventilation, and, as a compensatory mechanism, in most cases of severe metabolic acidemia.

CHANGES IN PLASMA BICARBONATE

Changes in the plasma bicarbonate of the blood depend not only on its rate of formation in the tissues, absorption through the G.I. tract and elimination through the kidneys, but also, of particular importance in acute situations, on its rate of destruction by blood acids. Plasma bicarbonate is usually formed or destroyed at relatively low rates. It usually requires hours or days by the usual mechanisms to have a significant abnormality in the concentration of plasma bicarbonate in the blood, in contrast to the changes of pCO_2, which could be very rapid and can take place in only a matter of minutes. However, the destruction of plasma bicarbonate in the body by acids could be a very fast phenomenon and it is of primary importance in dealing with critically ill patients with severe metabolic acidemia. In some cases of cardiovascular shock, severe limitation of cardiac output, such as would occur in some cases of acute myocardial infarction, or even in other metabolic abnormalities such as severe renal failure complicated by shock, the rate of production of lactic acid within the body is so high that very frequent replacement of plasma bicarbonate may be necessary to keep the patient alive. In a case of severe lactic acidosis due to phenformin intoxication we had to give over 1,000 mEq of sodium bicarbonate intravenously in less than twelve hours in order to maintain a pH that enabled the patient to survive. In cases of cardiogenic shock, we have given as much as 1,500 mEq of sodium bicarbonate in eight hours with the patient also surviving the acute situation. I wouldn't like to mislead the reader, however, in thinking that metabolic acidemia always needs that type of drastic action. As a matter of fact, most of the clinical situations can be corrected even without giving plasma bicarbonate, if we are able to reverse the basic process that caused the drop in plasma bicarbonate. The problem of the treatment of metabolic acidemia will be reviewed in greater detail later in the book.

In clinical practice, the most common cause of a drop in the concentration of plasma bicarbonate is the accumulation of acids in the body, either by excessive formation, ingestion, or lack of excretion. Respective examples of these three processes would be diabetic acidosis, aspirin poisoning and renal failure.

The plasma bicarbonate in blood can be increased by one of the following mechanisms:

1. Increased administration, such as when administering bicarbonate intravenously in cases of cardiac arrest;

2. Increased ingestion, as seen in some patients with peptic ulcer that may use large amounts of sodium bicarbonate as an antacid;

3. Increased reabsorption by the kidneys. Under normal circumstances, approximately 5,000 mEq of plasma bicarbonate are filtered in the glomeruli and reabsorbed in the tubules in twenty-four hours, while some 50 mEq of hydrogen ions are excreted, mostly as NH_4^+ and some probably as $H_2PO_4^-$. But changes in the pH of the blood and in the concentration of some electrolytes may alter this mechanism of reabsorption and secretion. One typical example is the case of chronic respiratory failure with chronic retention of CO_2. In such cases, because of the decrease in pH the kidneys are stimulated to retain more bicarbonate in order to compensate the excessive acidity. Another situation of increase in plasma bicarbonate frequently observed in clinical practice is that of increased reabsorption in the kidneys as a mechanism of compensation when the level of chlorides in blood have decreased significantly. These may be seen in cases of protracted vomiting and in prolonged use of diuretics.

I would like to emphasize that even if the knowledge of all the chemistry and physics involved in the processes of ventilation and acid-base balance of the body is quite sophisticated and deserves

Physiological Considerations About Blood Gases

the full attention of researchers in the field, the acquisition of the basic concepts necessary to make sound decisions in clinical practice is relatively simple. Confusing terminology has contributed significantly to complicate the problem. The following are a series of short paragraphs aimed at clearing some of this confusion and at reaffirming some of the basic concepts:

1. It should be clearly understood that pCO_2 and "CO_2 combining power" or "total CO_2" are two things completely different. pCO_2 is a measurement of how much CO_2 gas is dissolved in a liquid, and as such, is measured in partial pressure (mm Hg). On the other hand, the so-called "CO_2" obtained when ordering electrolytes in the chemistry lab is an indication of the amount of CO_2 that can be liberated from a sample of blood by titration and it grossly reflects the amount of bicarbonate. This is so because when destroyed by a stronger acid, bicarbonate will liberate considerable amounts of CO_2 gas. A high pCO_2 will tend to lower the pH while a high "total CO_2" tends to increase it.

2. *The base excess.* The base excess is an index of the total base of whole blood and it takes into consideration not only the plasma bicarbonate but the buffering capability of the hemoglobin and blood proteins. Some clinicians still use the values of the base excess in order to calculate the possible base replacement in a given clinical condition. The problem, however, is much more complicated than the use of a simple formula. This has been a very controversial subject in the medical literature. On the whole, we think that it has contributed more to confusion than to help the patients. Problems of ventilation and acid-base balance are best handled with the three basic measurements of pH, pCO_2 and bicarbonate alone, and we have decided not to use the concept of base excess in this book.

3. Even if some CO_2 is transformed into bicarbonate and vice versa in the blood, we would advise the clinician to disregard such process when interpreting a set of blood gases and deciding upon therapy. The basic concept is that for the most part the CO_2, as measured by the pCO_2, is a gas that contributes to the acidity of the blood, while the bicarbonate is a chemical substance that decreases the acidity of the blood. They should be considered separ-

ately as far as their processes of formation and elimination are concerned and one has to keep in mind that the influence of each one on the other is relatively small. pCO_2 has to do with ventilation. Plasma bicarbonate has to do with the chemistries of the blood. The two of them are basically independent. The relative amounts of both in the blood will determine what the value of the pH will be.

4. We must not forget that the most critical measurement is that of the pH. Correction of abnormalities of pCO_2 and bicarbonate should not be attempted without reflecting first on what such a correction would do to the pH. We will elaborate on this point as we discuss therapy.

OXYGENATION

Arterial pO_2 is the best indicator of the effectiveness of the lungs in transferring oxygen from the air to the blood. Oxygen hemoglobin saturation of the arterial blood and arterial oxygen content indicate better the availability of oxygen to the tissues. The relationship of arterial pO_2 to oxygen hemoglobin saturation is well established by the hemoglobin dissociation curve. But in some cases, such as when dealing with carbon monoxide intoxication, it is possible to have a very good arterial pO_2 with very low oxygen saturation. The oxygen content depends not only on the percentage saturation of the hemoglobin, but also, very importantly, on the amount of hemoglobin present. An anemic patient, even with a good pO_2 and a good oxygen saturation, may not be providing sufficient oxygen to the tissues. We will center our attention on the pO_2 since we are now mainly discussing lung function.

At sea level, the normal arterial pO_2 would oscillate between 80 and 95 mm Hg. Values between 70 and 80, even if representing some hypoxia, are seldom of clinical importance.

At which point a low arterial pO_2 should be corrected depends not only on its value but also on the overall clinical situation. When hypoxia can be easily corrected without danger of hypoventilation, we usually like to administer oxygen to all patients with pO_2's below 50. When the pO_2 is between 50 and 70 we will administer oxygen if the patient has symptoms or signs of hypoxia. With pO_2's above 70, administration of oxygen is seldom indicated.

Higher than normal pO_2's in the blood can be harmful, particularly in newborns and infants, when the central nervous system is more vulnerable because it is not fully developed. In the adult patient signs of damage to the optic nerve and retina have been identified in some cases but is less likely to occur than in children. Nevertheless, since pO_2's higher than 150 have little added therapeutic value, we usually try to keep the pO_2 of all the patients below 150 mm Hg.

The toxic effects of oxygen on the lungs are seen more frequently. It appears that concentrations of oxygen over 40% in the inspired air are potentially harmful and when possible they should be avoided. This point is discussed in more detail when reviewing the problem of respiratory distress syndrome of the adult. The dangers of high concentration of oxygen, even if given at small flows, in patients with chronic obstructive lung disease are discussed in the appropriate chapter.

The pO_2 and oxygen hemoglobin saturation of the mixed venous blood can be of some help in particular situations. We understand by mixed venous blood the one that is obtained, usually with a catheter, from the right ventricle or from the pulmonary artery. Low pO_2 and low oxygen hemoglobin saturation in the mixed venous blood indicates that the blood has been depleted markedly of oxygen in the tissues. If the arterial oxygen content was adequate, low oxygen content of the mixed venous blood will be an indication of increased oxygen consumption or decreased cardiac output. In the patient confined to bed most of the time the cause will be low cardiac output. The normal pO_2 of the mixed venous blood ($p\bar{v}O_2$) is between 35 and 40 mm Hg. $p\bar{v}O_2$'s of less than 35 mm Hg usually are an indication of significant decrease in cardiac output. When the $p\bar{v}O_2$ is less than 20 mm Hg the deficit of cardiac output is very pronounced.

This simple determination of $p\bar{v}O_2$ is at times more informative than a complete calculation of cardiac output because it better indicates whether or not the cardiac output is satisfactory for the needs of the patient.

When the patient is not in shock and the $p\bar{v}O_2$ is abnormally high, we are probably in the presence of a left to right shunt, an abnormal venous return or an increase in cardiac output. When the patient is in shock, a high $p\bar{v}O_2$ may also be present indicating that the so-called "high cardiac output shock" exists. In this condition, the blood flow through the vital organs is usually good even though the blood flow to the periphery may be drastically reduced. This may indicate central vasodilation and peripheral vasoconstriction. When the patient recovers from such a condition, there is often observed a dramatic change in the values of mixed venous blood and in the clinical picture. Together with improvement of the patient's clinical condition (relief of vasoconstriction, increased blood pressure, increased urinary output and improvement of the sensorium), there is usually a significant reduction of the $p\bar{v}O_2$. This is attributed to the fact that when the patient is relieved of his shock state the blood distributes more evenly throughout the body, which results in a drop of the value of the $p\bar{v}O_2$.

RELATIONSHIP BETWEEN BLOOD GASES AND ELECTROLYTES

The plasma concentration of the different electrolytes is very important in relationship to blood gases because:

1. Abnormalities in such concentrations can produce significant symptoms and even death. The dangers of hyper- and hypopotassemia to cardiac and skeletal muscle contraction are well known. Hyponatremia is a well-established cause of mental confusion and even convulsions. All these changes can impair ventilation significantly, particularly in patients who already have chronic lung disease, producing an increase in the pCO_2 of the blood.

2. Of all electrolytes, bicarbonate is the only one that will directly affect the value of the pH. However, there is an intimate relationship between bicarbonate and other electrolytes, and changes of the electrolyte balance may bring about a change in

the concentration of plasma bicarbonate, indirectly changing the pH.

Sodium bicarbonate is, then, the *link* between blood gases and electrolytes. There are no known symptoms attributable to a change in the concentration of the plasma bicarbonate by itself. Its importance is due to the fact that it is one of the two essential factors that determine the value of the pH.

In order to keep an ionic balance in the blood (positive versus negative charges), absorption and excretion of electrolytes is regulated in bowels and kidneys by complex physiological mechanisms. The two main negative ions of the blood (cations) are the bicarbonate and the chlorides. The main positive ion of the blood (anions) is the sodium. Calcium, magnesium, potassium, serum proteins and other chemicals all contribute to the electrical balance of the blood. If we identify independently sodium, chloride and bicarbonate, and lump together the proteins and the rest of the electrolytes, we could establish a relationship among them that approximately would stand as follows:

$Na = Cl + HCO_3 + 17$, where the three electrolytes are expressed in milliequivalents per liter and 17 is a number that represents the end result of combining the electrical value of the other electrolytes and of the proteins.

Since Cl and HCO_3 are the largest contributors of negative electrical charges to the blood, it is easy to see that when one of them increases, the body will try to compensate by decreasing the other, and vice versa.

A typical example of how changes in electrolytes may change the acid-base balance is the case of the patient who develops alkalemia after prolonged use of diuretics. What happens in such situations is that the plasma chlorides are lowered by the use of the diuretics and, in order to keep the proper ionic balance, the kidneys save bicarbonate. The increase in bicarbonate will be reflected in a higher pH. The opposite occurs in cases of chronic respiratory failure where a chronic increase in pCO_2 produces a drop in pH, which, in turn, stimulates the kidneys to save bicarbonate in order to bring the pH to normal. In a chronic stage there will be a normal or slightly low pH, a moderately high pCO₂ and a moderately high bicarbonate. As a compensatory mechanism, the chlorides decrease. In such a situation, it would be unwise to try to force large amounts of chlorides in order to normalize their value, because by so doing, the bicarbonate will be forced down to normal and, as a result, the high pCO₂ without similar increase in bicarbonate will produce a low pH.

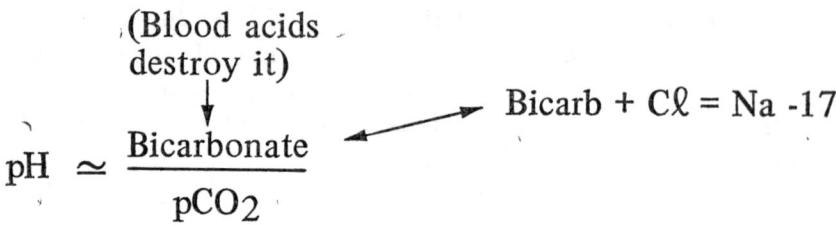

Figure 5. Relationship of Plasma Bicarbonate with pH, pCO$_2$ and electrolytes.

Figure 5 summarizes the basic relationships of bicarbonate to the Henderson-Hasselbalch equation on one hand and to the rest of the electrolytes and to the free acids of the blood on the other.

REFERENCES

Andrews, J. L. Jr.: "Physiology and Treatment of Hypoxia," *Clinical Notes on Respiratory Disease*. New York: American Thoracic Society, Vol. 13, No. 2, 1974.
Bartels, H. et al.: *Methods in Pulmonary Physiology*. New York: Hafner, 1963.
Bates, D. V., and Christie, R. V.: *Respiratory Function in Disease*. Philadelphia: W. B. Saunders, 1965.
Comroe, J.: *Physiology of Respiration*, 2nd ed. Chicago: Year Bk Med, 1966.
Comroe, J. et al.: *The Lungs: Clinical Physiology and Pulmonary Function Tests*. Chicago: Year Bk Med, 1962.
Crews, E. R., and Lapuerta, L.: *A Manual of Respiratory Failure*. Springfield, Illinois: Thomas, 1972.
Fenn, W. O., and Rahn, H.: *Handbook of Physiology*, Section 3, *Respiration*.
Filley, G. F.: *Acid-Base and Blood Gas Regulation*. Philadelphia: Lea and Febiger, 1972.
Lee, J. et al.: Central venous oxygen saturation in shock: A study in man. *Anesthesiology*, 36:472-478, 1972.

Petty, L. T. et. al.: The simplicity and safety of arterial puncture. *J.A.M.A.,* *195*:693, 1966.

Schwartz, W. B.: Fluid, electrolyte and acid-base balance, in *Cecil-Loeb Textbook of Medicine.* Philadelphia: W. B. Saunders, 1967.

Schwartz, W. B. et. al.: The response to extracellular hydrogen ion concentration to graded degrees of chronic hypercapnia: The physiologic limits of the defence of pH. *J. Clin. Invest., 44*:291, 1965.

Seldin, D. W., and Rector, F. C. Jr.: The generation and maintenance of metabolic alkalosis. *Kidney International, 1*:306, 1972.

Shapiro, B. A.: *Clinical Application of Blood Gases.* Chicago: Year Bk Med, 1973.

CHAPTER III

SYMPTOMS DUE TO ABNORMALITIES OF THE BLOOD GASES

HYPERCAPNEA

AN ELEVATED pCO_2 WILL PRODUCE vasodilation of the cerebral vessels and of the peripheral vessels. In the brain, the vasodilation is accompanied by cerebral edema and on occasions by papilledema. This is why patients with CO_2 retention very often experience very bothersome headaches. Through the mechanism of cerebral edema and the direct action of the high concentration of the CO_2, these patients become lethargic and finally may develop coma. Peripheral vasodilation is manifested by a warm and flushed skin, red and watery eyes, etc. Hypercapnea by itself can act as a significant depressor of the myocardium. It also decreases the affinity of hemoglobin for oxygen.

ACIDEMIA

A low pH will accelerate the transfer of potassium from the intracellular to the extracellular fluids, producing in some situations a significant hyperpotassemia. On the other hand, by the same mechanism it could bring to normal a potassium blood level which was originally low, masking the existence of an intracellular potassium deficit. Because of these possibilities, when acidemia is being corrected, close monitoring of electrolytes is indicated.

A marked drop in the pH can interfere with the action of sympathomimetic drugs. This is why an asthmatic patient who has already developed a significant degree of respiratory acidemia may not respond to bronchodilators until the pH has been improved. Through the same mechanism, acidemia may act as a myocardial depressant and may induce significant hypotension. A very low pH may even interfere with the conduction mechanism of the heart. This is why many terminal patients, in severe acidemia, develop bradycardia, prolongation of the QRS complexes, blocks and eventually cardiac standstill.

HYPOXIA

Low pO_2 will affect all the organs of the body, with its most dramatic effects being in the brain, the heart, the kidneys and the liver.

Hypoxia of the brain will produce mental confusion, and if severe enough, convulsions and coma. Hypoxia of the kidneys may result in impairment of the renal function. This is why renal failure is frequently encountered in patients with chronic respiratory failure. It is not unusual to find patients with chronic lung disease who at a time of decompensation have elevated BUN's and whose renal function improves with improvement of the pulmonary problem. Hypoxia of the liver may produce jaundice and other manifestations of liver failure. In patients with profound hypoxia we can observe at times signs of hepatocellular damage and even liver necrosis, with elevations of bilirubin, SGOT and SGPT, similar to what we may encounter in cases of cardiovascular shock.

Hypoxia of the heart causes depression of the myocardium and decreased cardiac output. In some cases it may increase significantly the irritability of the heart and may lead to fatal arrhythmias. Patients in acute, severe hypoxia will often show a combination of cyanosis, mental confusion, hallucination, tachycardia, hyper- or hypotension and profuse sweating.

Hypoxia is the most important cause of pulmonary hypertension and through this mechanism it may lead to the appearance of cor pulmonale and right-sided heart failure.

Finally, when the output of oxygen to the peripheral tissues is insufficient for the normal aerobic metabolism of the cells, anaerobic metabolism will take place, with production of lactic acidosis and rapid deterioration of the clinical picture.

HYPOCAPNEA

Low arterial pCO_2 is the most powerful cerebral vasoconstrictor known. In cases of hyperventilation, the blood supply to the brain decreases markedly as a result of reflex cerebral vasoconstriction. This leads to dizziness and eventually unconsciousness. It is well known to anesthesiologists that less anesthetic gas is needed during surgery when the patient is being hyperventilated. However, the cerebral hypoxia produced by the cerebral arterial constriction of hyperventilation is probably much more dangerous than the anesthetic gas itself and at present most anesthesiologists do not hyperventilate their patients.

Apparently, in order to have significant cerebral vasoconstriction as a response to hyperventilation and hypocapnia, the blood vessels should be healthy enough to be able to vasoconstrict. It has been shown experimentally that the amount of vasoconstriction as a response to hyperventilation is much more pronounced in young, healthy individuals than in elderly patients with advanced cerebral arteriosclerosis.

The clinical picture of the acute hyperventilator with sensation of dyspnea, increased alveolar ventilation, dizziness, numbness around the mouth and in the extremities and eventually fainting is well established.

When ventilating a patient with a mechanical respirator, hyperventilation is always a possibility and we should carefully monitor the blood gases and the mechanics of the machine. Inexperienced personnel may have a tendency to hyperventilate patients out of the belief that more of a good thing could not be harmful and also because a patient who is being hyperventilated is usually quiet without interfering with the mechanism of the machine. However, it is a mistake to hyperventilate the patients because of the potential cerebral problems that would occur due to brain hypoxia.

ALKALEMIA

When the pH of the blood is excessively high, significant abnormalities of the electrolytes can occur. Potassium is shifted from the extracellular to the intracellular fluid, resulting in hypopotassemia, with all its possible manifestations (muscular weakness, abnormalities of the myocardial contraction, EKG changes, etc.). The proportion between ionized and nonionized calcium may change, leading to tetanic convulsions. Alkalemia may be associated at times with low chlorides and low sodium, with its corresponding symptomatology.

It has been shown in some particular instances that a high pH by itself may induce a compensatory retention of CO_2.

HYPEROXYGENATION

Administration of high concentrations of oxygen has two potential harmful effects:

1. Damage to the lungs themselves. When high concentrations of oxygen are used for prolonged periods of time, with or without the respirator, the lung tissue experiences some structural damage. The severity of the damage is proportional to the concentration of oxygen and to the length of use. Figure 6 illustrates this point.

A particular problem is encountered with the use of high concentrations of oxygen during mechanical ventilation. Ventila-

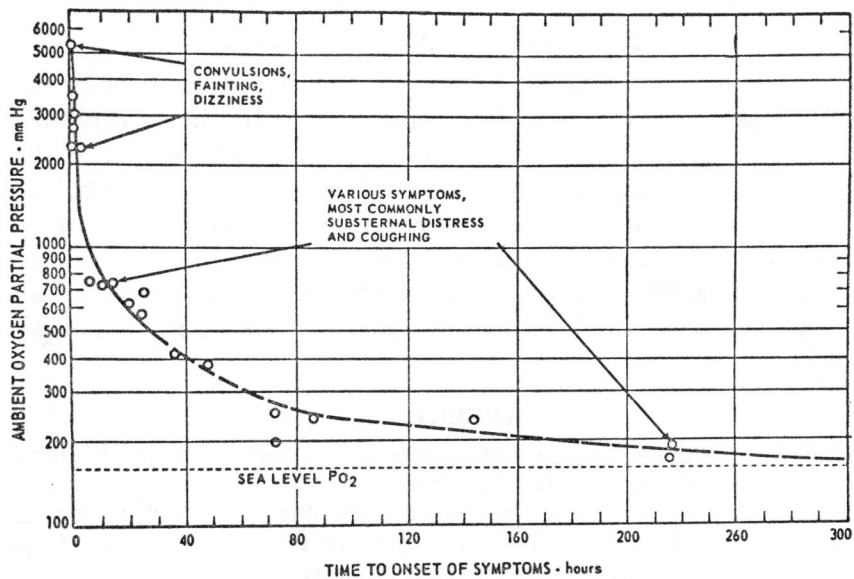

New England Journal of Medicine, 1966.

Figure 6. Onset of pulmonary signs of oxygen toxicity in relation to concentration of O_2.

tion with 100% oxygen should be avoided at all cost, if possible, because of the ease with which atelectatic areas may be formed in the lung. A part of the lung which is temporarily cut off from ventilation due to accumulation of secretions would maintain its patency if the patient is being ventilated with less than 100% oxygen, because the residual nitrogen will keep the alveolar spaces open. However, when pure oxygen is being used, rapid absorption of oxygen into the blood stream from areas cut off from ventilation would lead to alveolar collapse. Also, the direct damage of the high concentrations of oxygen to the lung tissue may produce more and more diffuse pulmonary disease, leading on occasions to what is known as "acute respiratory distress syndrome," which, in turn, would produce more and more hypoxia that will require higher and higher concentrations of oxygen.

2. High arterial pO_2's may be damaging to the central nervous system, particularly in its early stages of development. This is why high pO_2 is particularly dangerous in newborns. Please refer to the literature at the end of the chapter for more specific details on this subject.

COMBINED ABNORMALITIES

Most of the times, in cases of significant derangement of the blood gases, we do not find a single abnormality but a combination of several, and the symptoms and signs to be found in the patient will vary accordingly. Patients in acute respiratory failure who are not receiving supplemental oxygen will undoubtedly have the combined deleterious effects of hypercapnea, acidosis and hypoxia. Patients who have been hyperventilated mechanically, will present the combined symptoms of alkalemia and hypocapnea.

REFERENCES

Buttler, J.: Clinical problems of disordered respiratory control. Editorial. *Am. Rev. of Resp. Dis., 110:*695, 1974.

Comroe, J.: *Physiology of Respiration,* 2nd ed. Chicago: Year Bk Med, 1966.

Conference on the Scientific Basis of Respiratory Therapy. *Am. Rev. of Resp. Dis.,* Vol. 110, December 1974 (part II of 2 parts).

Ingram, R. H. et al.: Acid-base response to acute carbon dioxide changes in chronic obstructive pulmonary disease. *Am. Rev. of Resp. Dis., 108:* 225, 1973.

CHAPTER IV

GENERAL GUIDELINES OF THERAPY IN PROBLEMS OF OXYGENATION, VENTILATION AND ACID-BASE BALANCE

PROBLEMS OF OXYGENATION

THE THERAPEUTIC GOAL in cases of severe hypoxia is to improve oxygen content of the arterial blood to a point as near to normal as possible while at the same time avoiding the undesirable side effects of hypoventilation or oxygen toxicity. General considerations of oxygen therapy have been discussed in Chapter II. Details on how to deal with particular clinical situations can be found in the chapters discussing respiratory failure, mechanical ventilation, chronic bronchitis, pulmonary emphysema, asthma and respiratory distress syndrome in the adult.

Discussion of the mechanical means by which oxygen therapy is administered escapes the scope of this book. The reader will find them in the literature on respiratory failure, a sample of which appears in the biliography of this chapter. We would like only to offer at this point, in the form of "capsules," the following advice:

1. When administering oxygen therapy without the use of a mechanical ventilator, we must make sure that the oxygen is indeed reaching the patient at the desired concentration and flow. It is not unusual to find at times an oxygen delivery system apparently functioning well, with the oxygen bubbling through the water of the humidifier but, in reality, not reaching the patient because of a leak due to a faulty safety valve in the humidifier or because of failure to tightly screw the cup of the humidifier bottle. This is particularly true when the oxygen has to go

through an area of very narrow diameter such as the exit hole of some Venturi masks.

2. When using Venturi masks to deliver fixed concentrations of oxygen, there are in addition two significant points to be taken into consideration:

a. Total flow of gas through the mask should be a little higher than the average inspiratory flow of a patient. In a very simplified manner, if the average tidal volume is 500 cc and the average inspiratory time one second, the total gas flow in the mask should be higher than 30 liters per minute. The following formula gives the total gas flow when the O_2 flow and the F_IO_2 of the mixture are known:

$$\text{Total gas flow} = O_2 \text{ flow} \cdot \frac{0.79}{F_IO_2 - 0.21}$$

where both flows are measured in the same units, usually liters per minute, and room air is assumed to have an F_IO_2 of 0.21. (Table IV has been prepared with the above formula.)

TABLE IV

FACTOR TO BE APPLIED TO THE O_2 FLOW OF A VENTURI MASK IN ORDER TO OBTAIN THE TOTAL GAS FLOW OF THE MASK AT DIFFERENT F_IO_2 VALUES.

F_IO_2	Factor
0.24	26.3
0.28	11.29
0.32	7.18
0.35	5.64
0.40	4.16
0.45	3.29

b. The mask should be large enough to insure that an inspiratory flow faster than anticipated could be met by the total gas flow of the mask and the gas within the mask, without surrounding room air being drawn into the airways. In this regard the larger the mask, the more effective it will be.

3. When the nose and pharynx are being bypassed, such as it would be in administering oxygen to a patient with a tracheostomy or an endotracheal tube, care should be taken to ensure proper humidification and warming of the mixture of gases. Most

commercial "wall nebulizers," even when heated, are unable to heat the gas to body temperature when O_2 is being diluted with room air. Passing the mixture of gases through a "cascade humidifier" after dilution will solve this problem. Adequate temperature control should be maintained by placing a thermometer in the main tube past the "cascade."

4. IPPB treatments to patients who use a Venturi mask should be given with an F_IO_2 the same or only slightly higher than the F_IO_2 that they receive with the mask. The equipment used should be versatile enough to deliver the desired F_IO_2.

PROBLEMS OF ACID-BASE BALANCE AND VENTILATION

It is important to emphasize that the value of the pH is the primary consideration when looking into a problem of acid-base balance and ventilation. No one dies because the bicarbonate is high or low or because the pCO_2 is somewhat abnormal. Patients die when their pH is so abnormal that myocardial contraction and other metabolic processes in the body cannot take place. There are no known symptoms attributable to a change in concentration of plasma bicarbonate by itself. Changes in pCO_2 are indeed important, not only because of their influence on the pH, but also because of their influence in the circulatory system, and, in particular, the blood flow to the brain. But again, the most immediate danger to the life of the patient when the pCO_2 is abnormal stems from the possible changes of the pH. These considerations are the basis for a very important rule in acid-base therapy:

Therapy should be always directed toward normalization of the pH. Therefore, correction of bicarbonate or pCO_2 should only be undertaken if such a correction will result in a better pH. In other words: Do not do anything that would further deviate the pH from normal.

A good example is found in cases of Aspirin poisoning. Because the acetylsalycilic acid (ASA) destroys bicarbonate, the concentration of the latter in blood in the case of ASA intoxication decreases (hypobasemia). But at the same time, the ASA stimulates the respiratory center producing a considerable degree of central hyperventilation which in most instances overcompensates the decrease in plasma bicarbonate as far as its effect on the pH is concerned. A typical example of blood gases in a case of moderate ASA intoxication would be something like this:

pH 7.57, pCO_2 10 mm Hg, bicarbonate 9 mEq/liter, or

using the basic equation, pH ↑↑ = $\dfrac{\text{Bicarbonate} \downarrow\downarrow}{pCO_2 \downarrow\downarrow\downarrow}$

If we were to look at the values of the plasma bicarbonate only, it would appear logical to give an alkalinizing agent to bring the bicarbonate back to normal. But doing that in the face of central hyperventilation would be a mistake because, since we already have a high pH, additional bicarbonate or a similar substance would further increase the pH, perhaps to the point of being fatal. This is why in treating ASA poisoning, we should be guided primarily by the values of the pH and not by those of the plasma bicarbonate. In a more advanced phase of ASA poisoning, it is possible, however, to have a significant degree of acidemia because a so-called "ASA encephalopathy" could develop that would impair the respiratory center. If ventilation is impaired as a result, the pH will be dramatically low because there would be a respiratory and a metabolic component to the acidemia. In such cases, of course, assisted ventilation and infusion of plasma bicarbonate may be necessary.

A second rule of importance in acid-base balance and ventilation therapy is that, *if possible, the pH should be corrected by correcting the changes that made it to be abnormal in the first place.* As an example, if the pH of the blood is high as a result of overventilation with a mechanical ventilator in a case of respiratory failure, the logical thing to do is to decrease alveolar ventilation in such a way that will allow the pCO_2 to come up to normal so that the pH will also be normalized. The normalization of the pH could have been accomplished also by allowing the kidneys, given the time, to lower the concentration of plasma bicarbonate, but even if this would have produced a normal pH, it would have left the patient with two abnormalities to correct, low bicarbonate and low pCO_2. In a similar manner, a case of respiratory acidemia could be corrected by increasing ventilation or by administering bicarbonate. Obviously, the thing to do, if possible, is to improve ventilation because, by so doing, we normalize all parameters.

There are situations, however, when we must deviate a little from the above rules. An example would be some cases of severe respiratory acidemia in status asthmaticus. It is known that when the pH is very low, the catacholamines do not act effectively on the bronchial muscles and, in very difficult cases, we may be locked in a situation where bronchospasm persists, even when we administer liberal doses of bronchodilators. If mechanical ventilation also fails to solve the problem, it may be permissible in some instances to administer a little of sodium bicarbonate in order to temporarily bring the pH to a value where bronchodilators may be effective.

Therapy in ventilatory and acid-base balance disorders can be achieved by either direct or indirect means. A direct way of lowering the pCO_2 of the patient would be the use of a mechanical ventilator that by increasing the alveolar ventilation would enhance the removal of CO_2 from the blood. But in many situations, the same goal can be accomplished indirectly. If we can improve the condition of the airways and the well-being of the patient in general, we will be able on some occasions to allow the patient to improve ventilation on his own, therefore lowering the CO_2 by physiological means. We have found this indirect approach very rewarding in many cases of moderate respiratory failure. This problem will be discussed in more detail later in the book.

Similarly, we can change the concentration of plasma bicarbonate directly or indirectly. When a young diabetic in coma has a plasma bicarbonate of 1-2 mEq/liter and the pH is critically low, in spite of the presence of a marked hyperventilation, it is clinically sound to improve the acid-base balance by immediately injecting some sodium bicarbonate, without neglecting other therapeutic maneuvers. But once the initial emergency has been solved and the patient has been stabilized, adequate therapy of the diabetes itself with insulin, fluids, electrolytes and other measures, will create the appropriate conditions for the body to finish the correction of the acid-base abnormalities.

In the treatment of metabolic alkalemia we should consider

first the correction of the basic cause, the most frequent ones being the use of diuretics, extensive administration of bicarbonate, protracted vomiting, hyperaldosteronism and severe electrolyte derangement. When the basic cause cannot be entirely eliminated, or rapid correction is necessary, administration of chlorides should be considered. Potassium chloride should be used when the serum potassium is normal or low, or a different chloride compound when the serum potassium is high.

Metabolic acidemia should also be treated if possible by correction of its cause, but in cases that require rapid action sodium bicarbonate can be administered. When measurements of pH and pCO_2 are possible and sodium bicarbonate in injectable form is available, there is no place for the use of lactates in the treatment of metabolic acidemia. The drug Tham® offers no advantages over the sodium bicarbonate and can create more problems. In practical terms, sodium bicarbonate is the only drug to be used when active, rapid correction of metabolic acidemia is indicated.

The best indicator to decide how much sodium bicarbonate to administer in a case of metabolic acidemia is the blood pH. As a general rule, we advise the use of 50 mEq of $NaHCO_3$ for each 0.1 of pH below 7.3 in the average size adult. This dose is probably less than half the actual bicarbonate deficit in most cases. But repeating the blood gases in twenty or thirty minutes will allow us to see how much correction of the acidemia we have accomplished, and a second dose of bicarbonate can then be planned if needed. We find this conservative approach to the replacement of bicarbonate more practical than the calculation of the total base deficit for several reasons:

1. We should correct the pH, and not the deficit of bicarbonate. Correction of bicarbonate deficit regardless of the value of the pH could lead in some cases to catastrophic results if hyperventilation is maintained, as we have already discussed in the case of aspirin poisoning.

2. Present methods available for calculation of total bicarbonate deficit are not always accurate, because changes in the intravascular and extravascular spaces do not always occur simultaneously, and our calculations are always based on data obtained in the intravascular fluids.

3. Step by step correction of the acidemia is usually more prudent than rapid total correction. Total correction may result later on in severe metabolic alkalemia if the cause of the acidemia is also corrected. This is particularly true in cases of lactic acidemia, since the circulating lactic acid can eventually be metabolized back into bicarbonate.

Whether or not to use sodium bicarbonate in a particular case of metabolic acidemia, and how aggressively to use it, constitutes a medical judgment that should be made considering jointly the nature of the disease, the severity of the same, and the general condition of the patient. Table V shows the most common causes of endogenous metabolic acidemia, and some general guidelines of bicarbonate administration.

TABLE V
MOST COMMON CAUSES OF ENDOGENOUS METABOLIC ACIDEMIA, AND SOME GENERAL GUIDELINES OF BICARBONATE ADMINISTRATION

Renal	Mild	= No bicarbonate
	Moderate	= Oral bicarbonate
	Severe	= I.V. bicarbonate
Diabetic	Mild or moderate	= normally can be corrected without giving bicarbonate.
	Severe	= I.V. bicarbonate indicated
Lactic	=	bicarbonate almost always indicated, even in moderate cases. Close follow-ups of blood gases very important.

REFERENCES

Andrew, J. L. Jr.: Physiology and treatment of hypoxia, clinical notes on respiratory disease. *American Thoracic Society,* Vol. 13, No. 2. New York, N. Y. 1974.

Brackett, N. C.: An approach to clinical disorders of acid-base balance. *South. Med. J., 67*:1084, 1974.

Campbell, E. J. M.: A method of controlled oxygen administration which reduces the risk of carbon dioxide retention. *Lancet, 2*:12, 1960.

Conference on the Scientific Basis of Respiratory Therapy. *Am. Rev. of Resp. Dis.,* Vol. 110, December 1974 (Part II of 2 parts).

Garella, S. et al.: Severity of metabolic acidosis as a determinant of bicarbonate requirements. *New Eng. J. Med., 289*:121, 1973.

Kassirer, J. P.: Serious acid-base disorders. *New Eng. J. Med., 291*:773, 1974.

CHAPTER V

BLOOD GASES IN CHRONIC OBSTRUCTIVE LUNG DISEASE

GENERAL CONSIDERATIONS

WE SHALL START BY defining the concepts of respiratory insufficiency and respiratory failure. *Respiratory insufficiency* is the situation in which the pulmonary function of the patient is significantly altered, to the point of limiting his exercise tolerance, but still the patient is stable at rest and no significant damage to other organs of the body has occurred as a result of the limitations in pulmonary function. A typical example would be that of a person who has had a pneumonectomy in order to eradicate a carcinoma. The blood gases of this patient probably would be normal. He should be comfortable at rest, yet his exercise tolerance would be significantly decreased. In contrast, *respiratory failure* implies a more profound derangement of the function of the lungs. In a patient in respiratory failure, the blood gases are usually abnormal. The patient is hypoxic or retains CO_2, and as a consequence of either one or both, other vital organs are being impaired in their performance. Patients in chronic respiratory failure may have significant impairment of the function of the heart, brain, liver or kidneys, as a result of chronic hypoxia, hypercapnea, or acidemia. A more complete description of the signs and symptoms attributable to these derangements can be found in Chapter III.

Respiratory insufficiency is usually best assessed by pulmonary function tests. In the assessment of respiratory failure, we should consider not only the classical pulmonary function test, but also the blood gases and the general clinical picture. As a general rule, it has been suggested that we may consider a patient to be in respiratory failure when the pCO_2 of the arterial blood is higher than 50 mm Hg, or the pO_2 is lower than 50 mm Hg. This rule of the 50's can give an approximate idea but is by no means exact. General clinical evaluation is essential to complement the data obtained by the blood gases.

The treatment of respiratory failure due to chronic obstructive lung disease will depend not only on the degree of decompensation of the same but also on the basic process that is underlying it. In this sense it will be useful to differentiate between the three main causes of chronic obstructive lung disease: chronic bronchitis, pulmonary emphysema and bronchial asthma. We have to realize, however, that many times these components are intermixed in a particular case.

Chronic Bronchitis. Chronic bronchitis is characterized by a daily cough, with production of mucous sputum, for prolonged periods of time, and in the absence of a suppurative process that may explain the above symptoms. Early chronic bronchitis may be present without significant airway obstruction. However, patients with moderately advanced chronic bronchitis usually have airway obstruction. Most of the time the chronic bronchitis is also accompanied by some degree of bronchospasm. The blood gas picture in patients with chronic bronchitis varies from normal values in the incipient cases to very marked derangements of oxygenation and ventilation in advanced situations. When the distribution of the inspired air is sufficiently abnormal as to produce significant hypoxia, pulmonary hypertension occurs, and as a result, the symptoms of cor pulmonale may be present. Whether or not these patients develop retention of CO_2 depends not only on the degree of airway obstruction, but also on a variety of factors that affect the process of ventilation, such as the degree of mental alertness, general stress, degree of obesity, presence of electrolyte imbalance, other coexistent pathological processes (hypothyroidism, muscular dystrophy, etc.), and probably also to a great extent on the sensitivity of the respiratory center. There is clinical evidence to support the idea that some individuals may have a "hyposensitive" respiratory center, and would develop CO_2 rentention easier than the rest of the population. These are the patients who, if obese, may develop the so-called "Pickwickian syndrome," and in the presence of chronic bronchitis, they may be more prone to retain CO_2, falling into the category of "blue bloaters." In contrast, "pink puffers" would be patients with more forceful breathing but without significant hypoxia or CO_2 retention.

Pulmonary Emphysema. Pulmonary emphysema is characterized by the loss of lung parenchyma and pulmonary elasticity, which in turn allows the bronchial tubes to collapse, producing a significant degree of narrowing of the airways. As a result, moving the air in and out of the lungs becomes quite difficult and these patients have both an increased work of breathing and a marked decrease in their ventilatory reserve. A typical patient with moderately advanced pulmonary emphysema has forceful breathing with intercostal retraction and appears dyspneic even at rest. Since the caliber of the airways can be increased somewhat by keeping the lungs inflated, these patients usually adopt unconsciously an inspiratory position, bringing their tidal volume close to the top of their vital capacity. As a result, they usually have a smaller inspiratory reserve volume than normal and a larger expiratory reserve volume. Their vital capacity is decreased not because the total lung capacity is less but rather because the residual volume increases as a result of the trapping of air.

Patients with pulmonary emphysema could have at times a significant degree of clinical symptoms with shortness of breath and marked decrease of exercise tolerance, and still manage to maintain relatively good blood gases. It is not unusual to see patients with a one-second forced expiratory volume of less than 1000 cc and still having arterial pO_2 over 70 mm Hg with arterial pCO_2 within the normal range. However, as the disease progresses, invariably hypoxia appears. Even in patients with pulmonary emphysema who have practically no clinical signs of chronic bronchitis and who manage to maintain an arterial pCO_2 below 45 mm Hg, it is not uncommon to see their arterial pO_2 falling to values between 50 and 55 mm Hg at sea level, when their disease is so advanced that their ventilatory studies are decreased to values of approximately 25 percent of the predicted normal. In such cases, the hypoxia will produce pulmonary hypertension and signs of cor pulmonale may occur.

It is important to emphasize that patients with pulmonary emphysema but with little bronchitic component can remain relatively stable for years even in advanced phases of the disease. We have several patients who have remained stable for three to five years even though their one-second forced expiratory volume and the maximal voluntary ventilation have consistently been less than 20 percent of the predicted normal.

Bronchial Asthma. Bronchial asthma is characterized by paroxysmal episodes of bronchospasm accompanied by dyspnea and hypoxia. A typical patient of bronchial asthma will have no respiratory symptoms between attacks. He will have a marked decrease in his ventilatory studies and will be hypoxic at the time of an attack but his lung function will be close to normal when he is free of bronchospasm. Also, a patient with typical bronchial asthma does not cough when he is not experiencing an asthmatic attack. This point is valuable clinically to differentiate bronchial asthma from chronic bronchitis. A chronic bronchitic may have episodes of bronchospasm but even when he is free of such episodes, he would have a cough and some sputum production. Some asthmatic patients may develop with time a certain degree of chronic bronchitis. On the other hand, patients with chronic bronchitis and with pulmonary emphysema frequently develop bronchospastic attacks.

We should always keep in mind the fact that bronchial asthma is a potentially lethal disease. Many patients die every year of respiratory failure secondary to bronchial asthma. This is an area where therapy is usually effective and where with good understanding of the physiological abnormalities of the bronchospastic attack, combined with sound therapy, many of these deaths could be prevented.

TREATMENT OF THE CHRONIC OBSTRUCTIVE LUNG DISEASE

In treating chronic obstructive lung disease we should keep in mind not only that the patient's main problem is chronic bronchitis, pulmonary emphysema, or bronchial asthma, but also the degree of decompensation of the disease. Since the concepts of "compensated" and "decompensated" are somewhat vague, we shall define them as they are utilized in this chapter. By compensated, we understand the situation in which the patient is basically stable from day to day, even if he is having significant symptoms and significant abnormalities in his pulmonary function. A compensated patient is able to breathe without mechanical assistance, is conscious, and is in general able to care for himself even if he may need some assistance on occasions. In contrast, we understand by decompensated the situation in which the patient is rapidly deteriorating to the point that if energetic measures are not undertaken, he may be in danger of dying of hypoxia or CO_2 retention.

TREATMENT OF THE COMPENSATED PHASE OF CHRONIC LUNG DISEASE

Chronic Bronchitis. The general principles of therapy in chronic bronchitis include the elimination of pollutants from the airways (smoking, industrial and urban pollutions, etc.), facilitation of removal of secretions from the tracheobronchial tree, and treatment of bronchospasm. Some patients may require additional measures, such as occasional or intermittent use of antibiotics, use of steroids, and other medications or therapeutic maneuvers warranted by the clinical situation.

In general, newly diagnosed cases of chronic bronchitis in moderately heavy smokers do relatively well with very little therapy provided the patient stops smoking. We try to impress in our patients the absolute need to stop smoking. It has been our experience that with good counseling and with a clear explanation of the facts to the patient, most chronic bronchitics will stop smoking. The rate of success in having patients to quit smoking depends to a very great extent on the interest, understanding, and personal effort of the treating physician and reinforcement of this requirement by the other members of the health care team.

Since it is not our purpose to give a full description of all possible modalities of treatment in chronic bronchitis, we will discuss in detail only two points that are often controversial, namely, the use of IPPB (Intermittent Positive Pressure Breathing) and the use of oxygen.

IPPB and Chronic Bronchitis. Even if the administration of IPPB with bronchodilators is certainly beneficial in many instances, we should be careful not to establish a routine of giving this treatment to every patient with chronic bronchitis. We have seen patients improve remarkably with IPPB treatments, but we also have seen others who would develop an attack of bronchospasm every time that they would use the IPPB machine. In general, we like to have the following three conditions present before we advise the use of IPPB treatments to our bronchitic patients:

1. Actual need for inhalation therapy measures of this type. As we mentioned earlier, most cases of incipient or mild chronic bronchitis, and even some cases of moderately advanced disease, do well with the avoidance of tobacco and with the use of oral bronchodilators. We see no reason to subject these patients to the tedious daily use of a mechanical device and to the possible complications of the same.

2. We like to have objective and subjective evidence of improvement with the IPPB treatments before we decide to order them on a continuous basis. Objectively, it is a good practice to do ventilatory studies on the patient before and after the use of IPPB treatment with bronchodilators. Significant improvement in the ventilatory capability of the patient with treatment would indicate the presence of a significant reversible component of bronchospasm. These patients would potentially benefit from the use of such treatments.

3. No ill effects should be present after the use of the IPPB. This point is at times very difficult to evaluate. We should keep in mind, however, the possibility of the patient developing some of the following:

a. Some patients develop acute bronchospasm when the standard IPPB treatment is administered. The mechanism of production of the bronchospastic attack is uncertain, but we should consider the fact that with the standard method of applying the IPPB treatments, we are introducing a relatively fast stream of cold air into the bronchial tubes and that, on occasion, this could be quite an irritant. Also, bronchospasm can be produced by the use of some of the medications that have been advocated in different publications, but that probably do not have a place in the treatment of chronic lung disease, such as detergents, mucolytic agents, hyper- or hypotonic solutions, alcohol, etc. When we order an IPPB treatment we usually confine ourselves to prescribing a pure bronchodilator in an isotonic solution.

b. Since all bronchodilators have an ionotropic and a chronotropic effect on the heart, we should be mindful of the possibility of cardiac arrhythmia. This is particularly important in patients of advanced age who almost invariably have some degree of coronary arteriosclerosis. We have seen several patients who, in the course of receiving routine IPPB treatments, have developed atrial fibrillation and congestive heart failure, and who have improved remarkably with the cessation of the treatments.

c. The possibility of introducing infection to the bronchial tubes by contaminated equipment must always be considered. In this respect the degree of awareness and care of the patient and the family is very important, as well as the availability of sound instruction to them, either by the physician in charge or by competent respiratory care technicians.

d. We do not know to what extent the long-term use of IPPB treatments may be detrimental. In experimental conditions we have seen the tracheobronchial tree of laboratory animals develop signs of acute inflammation after the application of IPPB treatments. Recently published studies have reported the development of acute pulmonary edema in laboratory animals ventilated mechanically. However, we should consider the fact that the situation and indications are not the same in the experimental animal as in the chronic bronchitic, and that on the basis of the general experience of many physicians we cannot conclude at present that these treatments are detrimental.

The Use of Oxygen in Chronic Bronchitis. There is sufficient evidence to suggest that in cases of chronic bronchitis with significant hypoxia, the use of oxygen for several hours a day is greatly beneficial. Some studies suggest that fifteen hours a day of oxygen administration may cause a reversal of pulmonary hypertension in hypoxic patients. Arterial blood gases may be of great help in deciding which patient should or should not use oxygen at home. Arterial blood gases, however, should not be the only deciding factor. The presence of clinical signs of cor pulmonale or of other derangements secondary to hypoxia may be an indication for the use of oxygen even when the arterial pO_2 is not very low. As a general guide, it would appear that patients whose arterial pO_2 is better than 65 mm Hg would not benefit greatly from the use of oxygen on a continuous basis. On the other hand, patients with a pO_2 below 50 would almost always benefit from the use of oxygen. Patients with a pO_2 between 50 and 65 should probably be placed on oxygen only when significant symptoms secondary to hypoxia exist. There is a definite relationship between the level of hypoxia and the development of cor pulmonale. It is extremely unusual to find pulmonary hypertension on the basis of chronic lung disease when the pO_2 of the patient is still relatively normal.

The use of mixed venous pO_2 as an expression of the severity of tissue hypoxia is being advocated. We have found this measurement very helpful through the years in treating acutely ill patients in intensive care settings (see Chapter II), but its use in stable ambulatory patients appears to be impractical in most instances.

When using oxygen at home on a routine basis in the patient with chronic bronchitis who is significantly hypoxic, it is extremely important to do so in a way as to minimize the possibility of CO_2 retention. *Low concentrations of oxygen should be used.* We prefer the use of a Venturi type of mask that would give 24 to 28 percent oxygen.

Pulmonary Emphysema. Many of the things said for the treatment of the compensated phase of chronic bronchitis also apply to pulmonary emphysema, particularly if we consider the fact that most cases of pulmonary emphysema have a significant bronchitic component. However, in most instances the emphysematous changes of the lungs by themselves require little if any treatment. Emphysematous patients with little bronchitic component frequently do well without any treatment at all. These patients should be observed periodically and therapy initiated only when something treatable appears, such as infection, cardiac decompensation, etc. It appears that there is little or no advantage to the use of IPPB treatments in patients who are compensated, stable, and without bronchitic symptoms, even when the pulmonary emphysema is significantly advanced. What has been said about the use of oxygen in the treatment of chronic bronchitis also applies to pulmonary emphysema.

The use of physical therapy and of specific "breathing exercises" in cases of advanced pulmonary emphysema is debatable. There is agreement on the fact that a stable patient with pulmonary emphysema should try to remain active physically, within the limits of his tolerance. It is quite possible that the greatest benefit of the so-called "rehabilitation programs" of chronic emphysematous patients is derived from the fact that it allows for a better medical observation of these patients and encourages them to remain active physically, rather than from the specificity of the exercises used. Physical conditioning increases the efficiency of the muscles in the use of oxygen, allowing the patient to do more work with the same oxygen consumption. Slow, deep breathing with pursed lips may, on occasions, increase the arterial pO_2 a little. But there is no evidence in the literature at present to suggest that the learned patterns of breathing are used by patients in times of respiratory distress or that they contribute to prolong life.

Bronchial Asthma. It is not our purpose in this book to enter into a comprehensive description of bronchial asthma. A rational program of avoidance of pollutants and allergens, possible desensitization, use of bronchodilators, cromolyn sodium, and in some cases steroids, should be organized individually for each patient according to the particular conditions of the case. We would like to emphasize, however, the fact that bronchial asthma, particularly in patients of middle or advanced age, is on occasions a very difficult problem which, not infrequently, leads to acute severe respiratory failure. Because of this possibility, physicians treating patients with bronchial asthma should be knowledgeable in the details of therapy in acute respiratory failure or should have readily available consultants in this field.

We should keep in mind that hypoxia is a very well-established cause of bronchospasm and that when a patient develops status asthmaticus the hypoxia that invariably follows may be one of the factors that makes recovery difficult. In such cases, judicious and controlled use of oxygen, either by Venturi mask or in the mixture of gases that drive the IPPB machine, may be of significant benefit.

TREATMENT OF THE DECOMPENSATED PHASE OF CHRONIC LUNG DISEASE

A patient with chronic obstructive lung disease who enters the phase of decompensation, with increasing levels of arterial pCO_2, should always be treated in an intensive care setting. Direct observation of the patient at all times by trained intensive care personnel is mandatory. The details and degree of aggressiveness of the therapy will vary from case to case, depending on the particular condition. It is essential to keep in mind that these patients can deteriorate very rapidly and that mechanical ventilation may have to be instituted at a moment's notice. This is why an intensive care unit where these types of patients are treated should have at all times the facilities necessary for supportive ventilation, as well as the personnel capable of initiating and managing it.

In deciding when to start mechanical ventilation, a variety of factors should be taken into consideration:

1. *Progression of the decompensation.* A rising arterial pCO_2 after a sensible therapeutic regime has been established is usually an indication for mechanical ventilation. But, on the other hand, we may have patients who have chronically had a relatively high pCO_2 and who are able to function at that level of hypercapnea. In these patients usually the arterial pH will be close to normal because time has allowed for a compensatory increase in the plasma bicarbonate, whereas the patients with acute and progressive decompensation will have a low arterial pH as a result of the rising pCO_2 (respiratory acidemia).

2. *Other medical problems of the patient.* Patients with sig-

nificant cardiovascular problems, such as myocardial irritability, congestive heart failure, advanced arteriosclerosis, etc., may have to be treated more aggressively. Moderate degrees of hypoxia or acidemia may trigger fatal complications in these patients that would not be likely to occur if their cardiovascular system were intact.

3. *Degree of fatigue of the patient.* This is particularly important in cases of status asthmaticus. It is our observation that patients that have gone three nights without sleep due to the fatigue of the status asthmaticus are so tired that their will to fight for their breath is greatly diminished and they are much more apt to go into acute CO_2 retention. This is why we may intubate and treat with mechanical ventilation a patient with a mild to moderate elevation of CO_2 resulting from status asthmaticus when he has been deprived of sleep by the effort of breathing for considerable periods of time, whereas in another patient with CO_2 retention who has had his problem for only a few hours we may adopt a more conservative attitude.

4. *Previous history of the patient.* Knowing the patient well and having treated him during previous attacks of respiratory failure can give significant information to the physician. We have some patients who tolerate endotracheal intubation surprisingly well, with little discomfort, with little or no adverse effects. They remain alert during the entire process and require no sedation or restraining while the endotracheal tube is in place and mechanical ventilation is being applied. Some of these patients are so experienced in the treatment of their acute attacks of decompensation that they may even request, on occasion, the intubation. We may be more inclined to intubate and treat with mechanical ventilation one of these patients than someone who may be prone to panic and may require heavy sedation.

5. *Experience of the physician and respiratory care personnel.* This is a very important factor. With good experience in the treatment of these types of problems and with a first-class team of respiratory care personnel capable of expertly managing mechanical ventilation and its possible complications at all times, the institution of such procedure is safer and can be used more aggressively.

Many of the factors mentioned above are based on the characteristics of the patient, the experience of the physician and the degree of sophistication of the intensive care unit. It is difficult to give precise guidelines as to when the patient should be started on mechanical ventilation. As a general rule we institute the procedure when we see significant risk of the patient rapidly deteriorating without it. We have found through the years that as our respiratory teams develop and acquire more sophistication we have been using mechanical ventilation more. This does not mean that the possible complications of mechanical ventilation should be taken very lightly. A patient on a respirator is almost completely dependent on the alertness and knowledge of the personnel around him. A malfunction of the machine or an inadvertent erroneous maneuver may cause the death of a patient who otherwise may have had a better chance of survival if he had been left alone. A physician treating those types of cases should be mindful of all possible complications and has a great responsibility in developing and maintaining the skills of the personnel in the respiratory unit. Because of the turn-over of personnel that invariably exists in all units, a continuous educational program in respiratory care is mandatory.

Intubation Versus Tracheostomy. Once the decision to apply mechanical ventilation has been made, we have to decide whether to intubate a patient or to perform a tracheostomy. If intubation is chosen as the initial procedure, the decision also has to be made as to whether to place a nasotracheal or oral tracheal tube. In general, we always start with oral tracheal intubation. The advantages over a tracheostomy are obvious: rapidity of the procedure and absence of a surgical wound. Tracheostomy could be done later on if we see that mechanical ventilatory support will be necessary for prolonged periods of time. Nasotracheal intubation has its advantages and may be the procedure of choice when a very short period of mechanical ventilation is contemplated, such as during surgery. The tube is usually anchored more securely with nasotracheal than with oral tracheal intubation. On the other hand, the possibility of bleeding as a result of trauma to the nasal cavity is real and on occasions very important. We also have to be mindful of the possibility of pressure necrosis of the nostrils or of other structures of the nasal cavity. In advocating oral tracheal intubation we are only stating our own preference which is, in part, related to the fact that we have had more experience with such a procedure. The tube should be placed and secured in such a way that, considering the characteristics of the patient and the training and experience of the personnel around, a maximum of efficiency and safety can be achieved.

In deciding whether and when to do a tracheostomy in a patient already intubated we take into consideration the following points:

1. *The nature of the disease itself.* We have found that patients in status asthmaticus almost invariably can be handled well with endotracheal intubation and without tracheostomy. In the many scores of asthmatic patients that we have treated with mechanical ventilation in the past eight years, we had to do tracheostomy only in one case. The only two deaths that we have had among this group of patients have been the result of fulminating tension pneumothorax and pneumomediastinum, which probably could have occurred even easier with a tracheostomy in place. In general, an asthmatic patient in status asthmaticus does not need to be intubated for more than two or three days, and the tube is usually well-tolerated during this period of time. We should remember, however, that the development of laryngeal edema and stridor with complete obstruction of the airway is a very real possibility. When the endotracheal tube is being removed the patient should be observed attentively for the next thirty to sixty minutes, and we must be ready to reintubate the patient with a small tube should a laryngeal problem arise.

2. *The contemplated length of mechanical ventilation.* In general, we request a tracheostomy when we see, after four or five days of endotracheal intubation, that mechanical ventilation, continuously or intermittently, will still be required for longer periods of time.

3. *Training of the personnel in the intensive care unit.* If the personnel of the intensive care unit are not trained adequately in the care of endotrachel tubes, we may consider sooner the possibility of a tracheostomy. This is not to say that tracheostomy is free of complications and its care is easier. But, in general, the

complications with the endotracheal tube are more sudden and demand more immediate aggressive action (accidental extubation, kinking of the endotracheal tube, etc.).

REFERENCES

Barach, A. L.: Hypercapnia in chronic obstructive lung disease. An adaptive response to low-flow oxygen therapy. *Chest, 66*:112, 1974.

Chaves, A. D. et al.: Oxygen therapy in cardiopulmonary disease: A statement by the committee on therapy, American Thoracic Society. *Am. Rev. Resp. Dis., 101*:811, 1970.

Conference on the Scientific basis of Respiratory Therapy. *Am. Rev. Resp. Dis.*, Vol. 110, December 1974 (Part II of 2 parts).

Degre, S. et al.: Hemodynamic responses to physical training for patients with chronic lung disease. *Am. Rev. Resp. Dis., 110*:395, 1974.

Karpick, R. J.: Recent advances in respiratory therapy. *Med. Ann. DC., 43*: 137, 1974.

Nadel, J. A.: Mechanisms of airway response to inhaled substances. *Arch. Environ. Health, 16*:171, 1968.

Petty, T. L.: Systemic intensive respiratory care. *Chest, 65*:363, 1974.

Petty, T. L.: Does treatment for severe emphysema and chronic bronchitis really help? (A response) *Chest, 65*:124, 1974.

Petty, T. L.: Editorial. A critical look at IPPB. *Chest. 66*:1, 1974.

Symposium on Chronic Respiratory Disease. *Med. Clin. N. Amer., 57,* May 1973.

Waltemath, C. L., and Bergman, N. A.: Increased respiratory resistance provoked by endotracheal administration of aerosols. *Am. Rev. Resp. Dis., 108*:520, 1973.

Webb, H. H., and Tierney, D. F.: Experimental pulmonary edema due to intermittent positive pressure ventilation with high inflation pressures. Protection by positive end-expiratory pressure. *Am. Rev. Resp. Dis., 110*: 556, 1974.

CHAPTER VI

MECHANICAL VENTILATION

ONCE THE DECISION has been made to introduce an artificial airway and to help the patient mechanically with ventilation, a series of factors should be taken into consideration. We have to decide about the type of ventilator to be used, how to set it properly to adjust to the characteristics of the patient being treated and to keep always in mind that during mechanical ventilation the patient is completely dependent on our actions. We will review separately the processes of ventilation, oxygenation, humidification and temperature control during mechanical ventilation.

CHOICE OF VENTILATOR

The devices used to assist ventilation mechanically usually fall into one of the following categories:

1. *Pressure ventilator.* The flow of gas is initiated automatically or by the inspiratory effort of the patient and it is interrupted when the pressure in the system reaches a preset value.

2. *Volume ventilator.* The flow of gas is initiated as in the pressure ventilator but it is interrupted only when a given preset amount of gas has been delivered by the machine.

3. *Time and flow ventilator.* The gas is allowed to flow in each inspiration at a given flow rate for a predetermined period of time.

4. *Continuous flow.* Used mainly in children; in this type of respirator the air flows continuously from its source; inspiration is produced by obstructing the exhalation valve, thereby diverting the flow of gas into the lungs; at the end of inspiration the exhalation valve is open and the flow of gas from the machine and from the patient's lungs goes jointly out through the exhalation valve.

The different types of ventilators vary on the details described

Mechanical Ventilation 65

above and on many other technical features. However, their basic concept is always the same: a "Y" tube is attached by one of the ends to the source of gas, by the second end to the patient's lungs and by the third end to the exhalation valve. By appropriately combining flow of gas with closure of the exhalation valve the desired effect of intermittent inflation of the lungs is achieved. Detailed description of all the capabilities of the different ventilators escapes the scope of this book. The physician in charge of regulating mechanical ventilation should be, however, very much aware of all the technical aspects of the different ventilators.

More than the principle involved, it appears that the important factors in deciding about the type of ventilator to be used are mainly the versatility of the machine and the ability of the respiratory care personnel to understand and operate well a given ventilator. We decide many times on the use of a volume ventilator as opposed to a pressure ventilator, not because of the principle involved but because the volume ventilator may have the capability of having the gas flow and oxygen concentrations adjusted in a more exact manner. In general, almost any ventilator can handle almost any situation provided that there is sufficient skill, ingenuity and common sense applied.

VENTILATION

The adjustment of the settings of a mechanical ventilator is based primarily on the mechanics of ventilation in the particular case involved and on the values of the arterial blood gases.

Mechanics of Ventilation. Our aim should be to introduce an adequate volume of gas in the lungs of the patient with tolerable pressures. We should always keep in mind that in patients with chronic obstructive lung disease the expiratory phase is always prolonged, and that the ventilator is unable to accelerate the exit of gas from the lungs. This is why it is imperative that patients with severe obstructive lung disease be given a long expiratory phase when ventilating mechanically. A patient with very tight bronchospasm as a result of status asthmaticus will usually be ventilated well with tidal volumes of 700 to 1000 cc's if we allow five or six seconds for the expiratory phase (respiratory rates of 7 to

10 per minute) while we may be unable to introduce more than 300 cc's into the lungs of the patient, even with very high pressure, if we insist on having a respiratory rate of twenty per minute or more. Failure to keep these very low rates can create disastrous consequences. An asthmatic patient may require a peak pressure of 70 cm of water to obtain a tidal volume of only 300 cc's of gas when ventilated at twenty per minute and yet the same patient may accept 1000 cc's of tidal volume with pressure of no more than 35 cm of water if the rate is slowed to eight per minute.

Patients with chronic obstructive lung disease usually require lower inspiratory flow rates than the ones ventilated for other problems. Since the airways are narrow, they cannot accept a very large flow without creating turbulence. In order to find the proper setting, we usually start ventilating the patient with very low flow and keep increasing it little by little every three or four breaths. We stop increasing the flow when we see that further increase will create higher pressures in order to deliver the same tidal volume. In general, the average emphysematous patients are usually well ventilated with flows of around 45 to 55 liters per minute but in some patients with very narrow airways we have had to use flows as low as 30 liters per minute.

The conditions described above apply, as seen, to patients where the main problem is narrowing of the airways. In contrast, there are other patients who are ventilated because of severe parenchymatous disease but whose airways are more or less intact, and they need an altogether different setting of the ventilator. A typical case of parenchymatous disease without airways involvement is the so-called "respiratory distress syndrome of the adult." These patients will be described in more detail in another chapter. Briefly, they are characterized by heavy infiltration of the parenchyma with marked stiffness of the lung, marked increase in physiological dead space and severe hypoxia. These patients are better ventilated with very high inspiratory flows, at times as much as 100 liters per minute. Because of the marked increase in the physiological dead space they usually require large minute ventilation which is usually achieved by using large tidal volumes and relatively rapid respiratory rates of twenty to thirty per minute. Because of the generalized microatelectasis involving most of the lungs of these patients, the use of positive end expiratory pressure (PEEP) is necessary. Table VI summarizes the basic characteristics of ventilation in patients with airway disease as opposed to the ones with primarily parenchymatous disease.

TABLE VI
CHARACTERISTICS OF MECHANICAL VENTILATION IN PATIENTS WITH AIRWAY OBSTRUCTION AND IN PATIENTS WITH PARENCHYMATOUS DISEASE.

	Airway obstruction	Parenchymatous disease without airway obstruction
Inspiratory flow	Low	High
Tidal volume	Large	Normal or Large
Resp. rate	Low	High
F_IO_2	0.30 to 0.40	0.40 or more

Blood Gases in Mechanical Ventilation. pCO_2 and pH are the basic figures that we have to keep in mind when adjusting the ventilation of a patient on a ventilator. Plasma bicarbonate is important as it contributes with the pCO_2 to the final value of the pH. Oxygenation will be discussed separately.

Our goal should be to keep the pH and pCO_2 near normal values. When there is a conflict between both because of the existence of an acid-base abnormality, normalcy of the pH takes preference. As an example, if a patient has a normal pH, an elevated pCO_2 and an elevated plasma bicarbonate, as is sometimes the case in patients with chronic compensated respiratory failure, it would be unwise to suddenly lower the pCO_2 to normal values because this would in turn create a marked alkalemia which would be more dangerous to the life of the patient than the elevated pCO_2 by itself. Ventilation, thus, should only be changed in order to bring the pCO_2 closer to normal when by so doing the pH is also approaching a value closer to normal.

Since there is almost a direct relationship between the amount of minute ventilation and the amount of CO_2 being removed from the body, when correction of ventilation is indicated, we could use the following formula:

$$\text{New minute ventilation} = \text{old minute ventilation} \times \frac{\text{actual paCO}_2}{\text{desired paCO}_2}$$

Thirty minutes after ventilation is adjusted, new blood gases will tell us if further correction is necessary.

OXYGENATION

Since most patients being ventilated mechanically have some parenchymatous abnormality, acute or chronic, we will be using in most cases a concentration of oxygen higher than that of room air. In general, we should use the concentration of oxygen in the inspired air that would produce a normal pO_2, provided that by so doing we are not using high concentrations of oxygen for prolonged periods of time. It is generally agreed that a concentration of oxygen of 40% or less is usually not harmful to the lung tissue. Therefore, *we use whichever concentration of oxygen is necessary to maintain a normal arterial pO_2 provided we do not have to exceed 40%*. When even with 40% O_2 the patient still remains hypoxic, a compromise has to be reached. In general, we are satisfied with arterial pO_2's above 50 mm Hg in patients who are otherwise healthy and who seem to be tolerating those pO_2's well, and we try to use the lowest concentration of oxygen that would give us this safe arterial pO_2. This is very seldom a problem in patients with chronic obstructive lung disease because most of them, unless they have heavy parenchymatous damage, will obtain normal arterial pO_2's with relatively low concentrations of oxygen. But it becomes very significant and at times a difficult problem to solve in cases of the so-called "respiratory distress syndrome of the adult." In such cases we occasionally still have a significant hypoxia even when using 100% oxygen. But since we know that such a high concentration of oxygen is very detrimental to the lung tissue, we apply in those cases very strictly the above-mentioned rule of using the lowest concentration of oxygen that would give a pO_2 of 50 mm Hg. 100% oxygen is something that we particularly try to avoid in all instances because when this is being used we are exposing the lungs not only to the damaging effect of a high oxygen concentration but also to the fact that by not having any nitrogen in the inspired air, pulmonary atelectasis is more likely to occur.

HUMIDIFICATION AND TEMPERATURE CONTROL

We use in all cases of mechanical ventilation a "cascade humidifier" in order to deliver 100 percent humidity at body temperature. Control of humidity and temperature becomes very important because in patients with mechanical ventilation we bypass the nasopharynx, which normally would contribute to humidification and warming of the air. Provided that the temperature of the inspired air is not kept above the body temperature, there is no danger of overloading the patient with water because no more water is being introduced in the inspired air than is removed by the expired air. We should keep in mind, however, that with fully saturated inspired air at body temperature the so-called "insensible loss" of water through respiration is eliminated, and this fact should be considered when calculating the water balance of the patient.

PRACTICAL POINTS IN THE CARE OF THE PATIENT DURING MECHANICAL VENTILATION

Mechanical ventilation is a complex subject and does require at times not only a solid knowledge of the pulmonary physiology but also good knowledge of the mechanical ventilators, experience, and ingenuity. Without trying to cover all of the possible facets and potential complications of the same we will enumerate here in the form of "capsules" a series of points that may be useful to the reader.

1. *Know the equipment well.* There is no way to "trouble shoot" without knowing well the mechanics of the machine and the physical principles involved. This is equally important for nurses and physicians, who have a tendency to shift this responsibility to the respiratory care technicians.

2. *Patient should be observed constantly.* Alarm devices

should be a complement but not a substitute for adequate observation.

3. Be alerted to the *signs of sudden severe hypoxia:*
   a. Breathlessness;
   b. Cyanosis;
   c. Profuse perspiration;
   d. Hypertensive crisis;
   e. Sudden bradycardia or tachycardia;
   f. Electrocardiographic signs of ventricular irritability.

4. Be always on the alert for *possible ventilator malfunction.* The most frequent problems encountered are:

   a. *Sudden shortening of the length of inspiration.* Usually means obstruction. This will most likely be in the artificial airway but it could also be in the patient's bronchial tree or in the ventilator. In patients being ventilated with very high pressures we should be especially aware of the possibility of sudden tension pneumothorax that would also give this pattern of abnormality.

   b. *Sudden drop in the system's pressure.* It means that the air is leaking out of the system. Most likely causes are disconnection of the ventilator from the artificial airway, disconnection of two pieces of the ventilator, loose cascade humidifier, loose nebulizer, deflated cuff of the artificial airway or exhaustion of the gas supply that powers the ventilator.

   c. *Chest does not expand even if machine keeps functioning.* Most likely causes: Disconnection of equipment, accidental obstruction.

   d. *The respirator blows continuously* in a pressure-controlled machine. Most likely causes: Disconnection, large leak, malfunction of exhalation valve.

   e. *Sudden increase in pressure* in the volume-controlled ventilator. Most likely causes: Obstruction, sudden atelectasis or pneumothorax.

5. In an intubated patient, extreme care has to be taken to *avoid accidental extubation.* If the patient is confused or otherwise not in complete control of himself and with full cooperation, he should be properly restrained. The hands should be restrained

Mechanical Ventilation

in a way that they could not be brought up to the face. On many occasions the chest has to be restrained to avoid the possibility of the patient bending over and bringing the head down to where the hand is. See Figure 7.

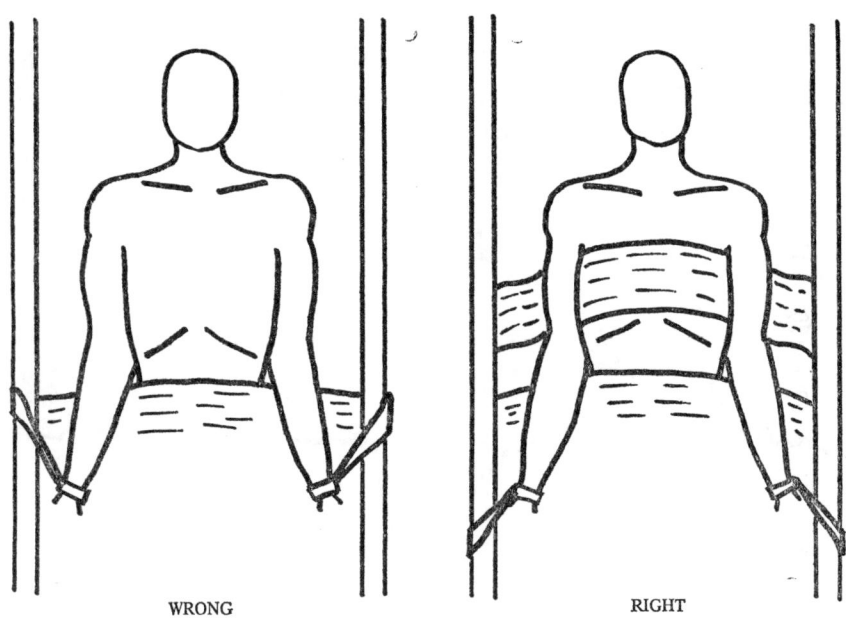

Figure 7. Restraining of an intubated patient to avoid accidental extubation. (a) Chest restrained with a folded bed sheet or with a jacket. (b) Hand restraints tied to bed further down, to avoid bringing hands to face.

6. *Intubation equipment should be readily available* to reintubate the patient in case of accidental extubation. Usually a tube slightly smaller than the one in place should be used for reintubation because of the possibility of laryngeal edema.

7. *Using the proper technique of endotracheal suction* is extremely important. Sterile glove and sterile catheter should be used every time. Suction should be extremely brief, particularly in patients with severe parenchymatous disease of the lungs. It is entirely possible to have the patient developing cardiac arrest due

to severe hypoxia when the maneuver of suctioning is prolonged for fifteen or twenty seconds. Figure 8 illustrates this point. In general, the cathether is introduced quickly and suction performed rapidly, the whole maneuver not lasting more than four or five seconds. If more suction is needed the patient should be given a few breaths with the ventilator and then suction is repeated. In cases of extreme hypoxia and severe parenchymatous disease of the lungs it may be wise to ventilate the patient with 100% oxygen for the three or four minutes prior to suctioning.

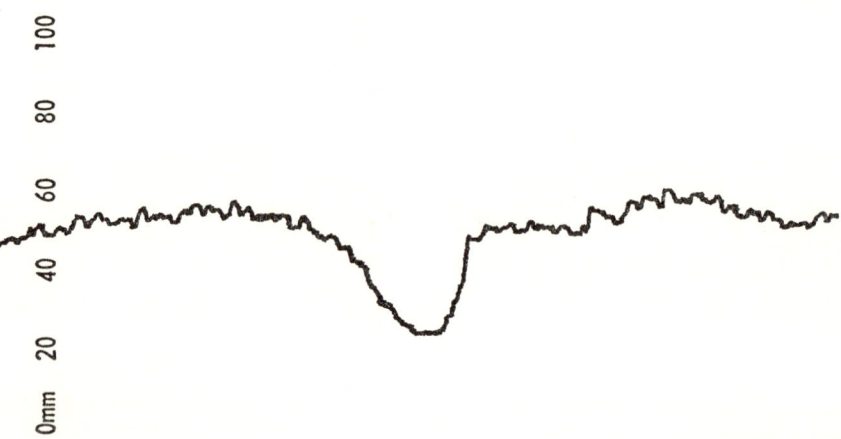

Figure 8. Arterial pO_2 of a patient on mechanical ventilation as measured continuously with an intraarterial electrode. Deep and prolonged hypoxia followed each suctioning maneuver.

8. It is recommended by the Center of Communicable Diseases that the *tubes of the ventilator be changed every twelve hours*. The cascade should be changed every twenty-four hours.

9. *Inflation of cuffs*. Soft cuffs should be used. The amount of air needed to inflate a cuff varies from patient to patient. We should use the smallest amount of air that would allow the ventilator to function effectively. A small air leak around the cuff is desirable in most instances providing that the ventilator still is working efficiently. The cuff should be deflated periodically. As a

general rule, this should be done once every hour.

10. *Positioning of tracheostomy tubes.* Care should be taken not to distort the position of the tracheostomy tube as a result of the pressure or the pulling of the ventilator. The suction cathether should enter the trachea freely. The position of the tube should change little or not at all when connecting the ventilator to it.

11. *Positioning and anchoring of endotracheal tube.* The tip of the endotracheal tube should be well above the carina. Once the right position is obtained and proven by X-ray, it is helpful to cut away the excess of endotracheal tube protruding from the mouth or nose and to leave between one-half inch and 1 inch of tube protruding from the level of the lips. By having a fixed distance protruding out of the mouth or the nose it is easier to maintain the proper position of the tube. Patients with teeth should have an oral pharyngeal airway to prevent biting of the tube. Figure 9 illustrates an effective way of maintaining the airway and the tube both in place. Edentulous patients many times would do well without the oral pharyngeal airway but in some cases, particularly when they use their tongue to push the tube out, the airway may be necessary.

12. *Adequate gastric intake* is advisable in patients on respirators in order to maintain proper nutrition, prevent the formation of stress ulcers and facilitate maintenance of adequate water and electrolyte balance. We introduce a nasogastric tube in most patients shortly after intubation. Once the endotracheal tube is in place at times it may be a little difficult to introduce a nasogastric tube. We have had better results by using relatively large N-G tubes and by guiding the tip of the tube to the opening of the esophagus, if necessary, with a finger introduced into the oropharynx. Antacids are used at regular intervals, usually every three or four hours.

13. Special attention should be paid to proper nutrition of the patient, and in particular their *level of plasma albumin* should be watched carefully. Many of these patients, particularly if they have been on a ventilator for a long period of time or if they develop the respiratory failure after a debilitating disease,

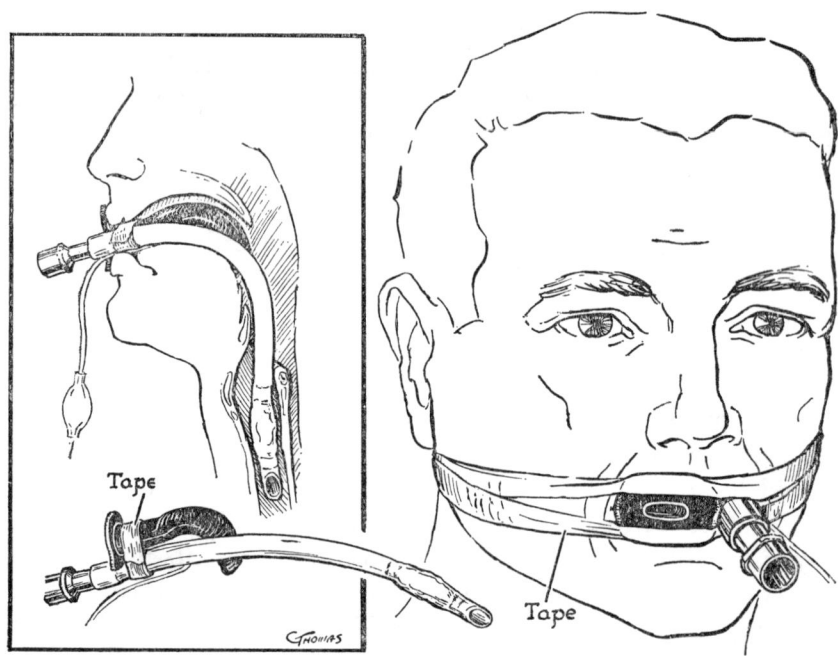

Figure 9. Maintaining endotracheal tube and oral airway in place in an intubated patient: endotracheal tube is taped to airway; airway is taped to face and neck.

may have very low plasma albumin. This, in turn, would facilitate the extravasation of fluid in the interstitial spaces of the lungs and would make the process of ventilation and the weaning of the patient from the ventilator more difficult. Albumin should be replaced intravenously when indicated. Cases of pneumocystis carinii pneumonia in patients receiving immunosuppressive drugs are particularly difficult in this respect. These patients usually have a very rapid turnover of albumin and it is not unusual to have to inject as much as 200 cc's of 25% human albumin daily for several days in order to maintain an adequate level of plasma albumin. The dosage should be adjusted individually according to the results obtained.

14. *Frequent cultures* should be obtained from the endotracheal secretions and the patient treated according to the results.

THE PROCESS OF WEANING THE PATIENT FROM MECHANICAL VENTILATION

There are no specific rules that could be given in order to discontinue mechanical ventilation. We should use our own judgement in every instance according to the characteristics of the case, previous experience of the physician in charge and skills of the personnel that will be observing the patient continuously in the intensive care unit. In general, we do not remove the endotracheal tube until we have had twenty-four hours of stable clinical situation with the patient still having the endotracheal tube but without receiving mechanical assistance other than a few minutes every hour. The use of CPAP (Continuous Positive Ambient Pressure) has been advocated in some situations, particularly in postoperative cases when the possibility of atelectasis has to be entertained. In cases of chronic obstructive lung disease the use of CPAP may in many instances add to the work of breathing without really bringing any benefits. Intermittent Mandatory Ventilation (IMV), with or without CPAP, may be indicated on occasions.

REFERENCES

Benditen, H. H.: Rational ventilator modes for respiratory failure. *Crit. Care Med.*, 2:225, 1974.

Chusid, E. L. et al.: Application of ventilators in acute respiratory failure. *Med. Clin. N. Amer.*, 57:1551, 1973.

Franklin, W.: Treatment of severe asthma. *New Eng. J. Med.*, 290:1469, 1974.

Gruzman, A. B. et al.: Special devices for supportive artificial pulmonary ventilation. *Biomed. Eng.*, 7:166, 1974.

McMahon, S. M. et. al.: Positive end-expiratory airway pressure in severe arterial hypoxemia. *Am. Rev. Resp. Dis.*, 108:256, 1973.

Meyer, J. A.: Mechanical support of respiration. *Surg. Clin. N. Amer.*, 54:1115, 1974.

Powers, S. R.: The use of positive-end-expiratory pressure (PEEP) for respiratory support. *Surg. Clin. N. Amer.*, 54:1125, 1974.

Zwillich, C. W. et al.: Complications of assisted ventilation. *Amer. J. Med.*, 57:161, 1974.

CHAPTER VII

BLOOD GASES IN ACUTE PULMONARY EDEMA

ACUTE PULMONARY EDEMA is one of the situations in which the importance of adequate ventilation, oxygenation and acid-base balance control is more dramatically shown. Even though acute pulmonary edema can be seen in cases of drowning, metabolic acidosis, septicemia, trauma to the chest, inhalation of toxic gases, and a number of other clinical conditions, by far the most common cause of pulmonary edema in clinical practice is the sudden failure of the left ventricular function.

In pulmonary edema, the interstitial spaces of the lung are engorged with fluid, the alveolar spaces become flooded, the bronchial muscles constrict and, eventually, the tracheobrochial tree fills with foamy fluid. As a result of these changes, the transfer of oxygen is impaired and hypoxia results. As the disease progresses, ventilation becomes difficult, resulting in CO_2 retention and respiratory acidemia. As the pH of the blood and the oxygen content decrease, the cardiac muscle becomes more and more inefficient, resulting in more pulmonary edema and poor cardiac output. Eventually, the peripheral tissues receive less oxygen than minimally required for the aerobic metabolism and production of lactic acid results, adding a factor of metabolic acidemia to the already acidemic blood. The end result may be asystole and death.

Clinically, during the initial hypoxic stage, we usually observe an anxious patient, struggling for breath, breathing against increased resistance, but actually hyperventilating. He is cyanotic, often perspiring profusely. On auscultation, we can hear scattered rhonchi, wheezes and basilar crepitant rales. The electrocardiogram usually shows some degree of tachycardia, diffuse myocardial ischemia, on occasions some premature contractions. As the disease progresses to the point of hypoventilation, or hypercapneic phase, the patient seems to be quieter, becoming mentally confused and eventually unconscious. Auscultatory sounds decrease drastically because of the decrease in ventilation. The eyes become reddish and watery. The cyanosis deepens. Pink, foamy sputum is frequently observed.

As the patient enters the phase of metabolic acidemia, events usually develop very rapidly towards a fatal outcome. Unconsciousness is profound. The breath sounds become markedly reduced. The heart rate usually slows. Pupils become pinpoint and eventually start dilating. The electrocardiogram shows wide QRS complexes with tall and "lazy" T waves, the rate decreases. Finally, the heart stops in electrical standstill, as the pH of the blood decreases to the point of making the electrical conduction impossible. In some cases hypoxia is so severe that it induces marked myocardial irritability, and ventricular fibrillation occurs preceding the standstill. This is more frequently seen in patients who have been treated with Digitalis during the acute phase.

TABLE VII
CHANGES OF VENTILATION, OXYGEN AND ACID-BASE BALANCE IN FATAL ACUTE PULMONARY EDEMA.

	pO_2	pH	pCO_2	Bicarbonate
Phase I	↓↓	↑	↓	Unchanged
Phase II	↓↓↓	↓	↑	Unchanged
Phase III	↓↓↓↓	↓↓↓	↑↑	↓↓

Table VII summarizes the above described phases of the natural history of fatal acute pulmonary edema.

The therapeutic approach to the acute pulmonary edema is twofold.

1. Correction of the oxygen, ventilation and acid-base balance abnormalities.

2. Measures directed toward the improvement of the hemodynamic conditions, such as use of diuretics, cardiotonics, etc.

In treating pulmonary edema, we must place in the proper perspective all the information obtained from examination of the patient and we must weigh carefully the benefits and potential dangers of the different therapeutic maneuvers. Therapeutic measures should be applied as the situation requires, keeping always in mind the possibility of iatrogenic effects. We think that it is highly inappropriate to resort to a routine of therapeutic measures where the name "pulmonary edema" automatically brings forth a battery of maneuvers, such as administration of Digitalis, diuretics, rotating tourniquets, etc. On the contrary, each patient should be assessed in his own situation and therapy directed in an intelligent manner.

Inhalation Therapy Measures and Correction of Acid-Base Balance Disorders. These measures should be applied in a gradual manner, depending on the particular phase of the pulmonary edema. Table VIII summarizes our approach.

TABLE VIII

THERAPEUTIC APPROACH TO ACUTE PULMONARY EDEMA FROM THE POINT OF VIEW OF RESPIRATORY CARE.

Phase I	=	High $F_I O_2$ by nasal cannula, Venturi mask or IPPB.
Phase II	=	Mechanical ventilation with high $F_I O_2$. Some patients may do well with mouth piece or face mask; some may require intubation.
Phase III	=	Mechanical ventilation with high $F_I O_2$. Intubation almost always necessary. Administration of plasma bicarbonate indicated.

During the hypoxic stage, administration of adequate oxygen by cannula or mask may be sufficient. This may be supplemented by the use of intermittent positive pressure breathing with high concentrations of oxygen. It is quite rewarding to see how this anxious and very distressed patient, who may initially have a slight difficulty in using the IPPB machine if he never used it before, experiences dramatic improvement in only a few minutes of IPPB use. In many cases, his perspiration stops, his breathing is considerably eased and he becomes calm, comfortable and often amazed at the rapidity of his recovery. The IPPB can be used in this phase with a mouthpiece or with a face mask. Most cases of acute pulmonary edema will not require anything more energetic. High flows in the respirator are desirable if the patient does not have chronic obstructive disease of the lungs.

In the phase of hypoventilation and hypercapnea, a more persistent and energetic approach to mechanical ventilation is needed. Some patients may do well with continuous use of IPPB with mouthpiece if they are conscious and cooperative. But in the most distressed patients, endotracheal intubation and mechanical ventilation is often needed. Once the patient is intubated, sedation can be accomplished and aspiration of bronchial secretions is facilitated. We should emphasize that even if aspiration of bronchial secretions is very important, this maneuver must always relinquish first place to ventilation. When a patient is intubated in a dire emergency, we should not waste time by trying to suction the patient persistently before applying mechanical ventilation. On the contrary, ventilation with high oxygen content should be done first. It is possible to ventilate a patient in acute pulmonary edema, even if he has an abundance of secretions in the tracheobronchial tree, provided that the right kind of equipment and the necessary know-how are available. After several minutes of mechanical ventilation, we can safely start to suction.

In the phase of metabolic acidemia, the above measures should be supplemented by correction of the bicarbonate deficit by intravenous injection of sodium bicarbonate. We should follow in this regard the general guidelines of the treatment of lactic acidemia, outlined in Chapter IV.

Diuretics. A diuretic of rapid action is indicated in acute pulmonary edema. Furosemide seems to be the drug of choice at present, not only because of its rapid diuretic effects, but also because it has been shown to decrease the venous return to the right heart, therefore, decreasing the overload of the heart almost immediately. 40 mg of furosemide intravenously or intramuscularly is our dosage of choice. If further diuresis seems to be needed, we would have to be alert to the possibility of electrolyte imbalance.

Digitalis. A fast-acting Digitalis preparation is used by most physicians in the acute phase of pulmonary edema in patients who have not been previously digitalized. We think that, however, before giving a dose of Digitalis to a patient in acute pulmonary edema, we should keep in mind the following:

1. Extreme caution should be exerted not to give an excessive dose. A patient who has been already digitalized, has a good chance of experiencing some of the effects of Digitalis intoxication when

he goes into acute pulmonary edema just because of the appearance of hypoxia and acid-base abnormalities that make the myocardium more irritable. The "extra push" of Digitalis that we see used at times in patients with acute pulmonary edema, who were already fully digitalized, is in our view particularly hazardous and we would not recommend it.

2. We should be modest in our expectation of therapeutic results attributable to the Digitalis in acute pulmonary edema. In severe pulmonary edema, the main therapeutic tool is not Digitalis, but the correction of oxygen and acid-base abnormalities, along with the positive pressure breathing and the reduction of venous return to the heart. We do not use Digitalis in treating a case of acute severe pulmonary edema because we think that the problem is best controlled by other means and the addition of the Digitalis drug may create more complications than may solve problems.

Sedation. Most textbooks advise that morphine should be administered in the initial phase of treatment of pulmonary edema, the reason given being that correction of the anxiety should help the overall clinical picture and that morphine, in addition, decreases the venous return to the heart. We have very serious reservations to the use of such a routine in every case of pulmonary edema. In the first place, patients in acute pulmonary edema have a good reason to be anxious. They are struggling for their life with their very labored breathing. They need to be extremely alert to keep the fight for breath. We very often see the anxiety disappear when successful treatment relieves their problem. Also, morphine or any other sedative drug will undoubtedly decrease the respiratory drive and may precipitate a progression of the condition from the hypoxic to the hypercapneic phase. Thirdly, the decrease in venous return obtained by morphine can be accomplished by other means, such as the use of furosemide, without interfering with respiratory drive and the state of consciousness of the patient.

Because of the reasons stated above, we have great reservations about the use of morphine in pulmonary edema. It is quite possible that tradition and incomplete observation may have played a significant role in the perpetutation of the use of morphine as a standard measure in the treatment of pulmonary edema. It is very probable that the patients helped by the use of morphine are usually the ones that are in the early stages of the hypoxic stage, without hypoventilation, who would get well anyway with the application of the other measures described above and without the use of morphine. It is our view that the blanket use of morphine in all cases of pulmonary edema, without adequate control of ventilation, oxygenation and acid-base balance, may be dangerous in most of the severe cases of this condition. On the other hand, we would not oppose its judicious use in very small doses in patients who are quite stable, provided that there is continuous observation of the patient by qualified individuals who would be able to start mechanical ventilation immediately should the need arise.

Other Supportive Measures, such as correction of hypopotassemia when present, correction of other electrolyte disturbances, etc., should be undertaken following the sound principles of intensive medicine.

It is interesting to see that the definition of pulmonary edema by Laenec in the early 19th Century already offered a very intelligent insight into the nature of the problem, as well as into the logical way of treating it: "Edema of the lung is the infiltration of serum into the substance of the organ, in such degree as evidently to diminish its permeability to air, in respiration."

REFERENCES

Aberman, A., and Fulop, M.: The metabolic and respiratory acidosis of acute pulmonary edema. *Ann. Int. Med.,* 76:173, 1972.

Avery, W. G. et al.: The acidosis of pulmonary edema. *Am J Med.,* 48: 320, 1970.

Ayres, S. M.: Ventilatory management in acute pulmonary edema. *Am. J. Med.,* 54:558, 1973.

Laenec, R. T. H.: *A Treatise of the Disease of the Chest.* London: Trans J. Forbes, 1932.

Miller, A. et al.: Acute, reversible respiratory acidosis in cardiogenic pulmonary edema. *J.A.M.A.,* 216:1315, 1971.

Miller, W. F., and Sproule, B. J.: Studies on the role of intermittent inspiratory positive pressure oxygen breathing in the treatment of pulmonary edema. *Dis. of Chest.,* 35:469, 1959.

Staub, N. C.: Pulmonary edema. *Physiol. Rev.,* 54:678, 1974.

CHAPTER VIII

BLOOD GASES IN CARDIAC ARREST

CARDIC ARREST, as we ordinarily see it in an acute care hospital, is usually due to one of the following causes:

1. Sudden arrhythmia that leads to ventricular fibrillation. These are cases with increased myocardial irritability, such as acute myocardial infarction, Digitalis intoxication, severe hypoxia, etc.

2. Acute impairment of ventilation leading to hypoxia and acidemia. Examples: Drowning, aspiration, etc.

3. Chronic progressive hypoventilation leading to hypoxia, hypercapnea, and acidemia, such as status asthmaticus, progressive respiratory failure, some cases of cerebrovascular accident, etc.

4. The so-called "metabolic acidemia" which we may see in cases of lactic acidemia (low cardiac output of the acute myocardial infarction, septic shock, hypovolemic shock due to hemorrhage or dehydration, etc.) or in other situations such as juvenile diabetic coma, advanced renal failure, ingestion of acids, etc.

5. A variety of derangements of the chemistries of the blood that make the heart irritable or the cardiac contraction impossible. The basic causes can be multiple, but the immediate cause of the cardiac arrest would be an abnormality in the chemistry of the blood, such as hypercalcemia, hyperpotassemia, etc.

The treatment of cardiac arrest will depend to a great extent on what the causative problem has been. No simple routine will constitute optimal treatment in all cases. We must be as objective and knowledgeable as possible in order to see all facets of the acute problem and treat them correctly. We will review in this chapter, however, some of the basic principles that apply to many of the cardiac arrests, with particular emphasis on the contribution of the determination of the blood gases and pH to the understanding and management of the acute situation.

Retrospective analysis of the deaths which occurred in a large general hospital indicates that even if the more dramatic cases are those of sudden arrhythmia, particularly in intensive care units, by far the most frequent cause of death is progressive deterioration of vital functions, such as ventilation, oxygenation and adequate cardiac output. In the hospital that we surveyed, approximately 50 percent of the medical deaths occurred in regular rooms and 50 percent in the intensive care areas. Most of the deaths in the regular rooms were in cases where aggressive therapy had been ruled out on sound medical grounds, but a given number of them occurred in patients that had a relatively rapid deterioration through a short period of time and who could have benefited by intensive therapy. We have every reason to believe that the same situation exists in most hospitals. This emphasizes the importance of having the nursing staff and the house medical staff as well trained as possible in the recognition of signs of acute decompensation of the vital functions. We think that the medical staff of the hospital has the duty of devoting a great effort to the continuous training of the nursing personnel, since it is usually a nurse who first recognizes the signs of a patient in distress.

A heart usually stops pumping in one of the following manners:

1. Sudden asystole.
2. Ventricular fibrillation.
3. Progressive bradycardia, followed by asystole.

Even with the acknowledgement that some exceptions exist, a general approach to these three modalities of cardiac arrest can be attempted as follows:

1. *Sudden asystole,* without previous warning, is usually the result of a conduction problem and the treatment is usually pharmacological (Atropine®, sympathomimetic drugs, etc.). Abnormalities in the blood chemistry may also be responsible for sudden asystole (hypercalcemia, hyperpotassemia, etc.) and adequate corrections would have to be made. Ventilation, oxygenation and acid-base balance problems become of vital importance when the asystole lasts for more than a few seconds. Abnormalities encountered in these parameters would have to be promptly and efficiently corrected. However, in most instances, supportive ventilation with a face mask and a bag, along with adequate oxygenation would be all that is required in short periods of asystole. It is wise to check

the blood gases after the acute problem is over, because of the possible abnormalities that may have occurred during the short period of asystole and because we should rule out previous unsuspected abnormalities of ventilation, oxygenation and acid-base balance that may have been contributing factors to the asystole.

2. *Ventricular fibrillation* is usually a result of excessive myocardial irritability. Hypoxia and acidemia may be very significant contributing factors in some of the cases, but more often than not, the basic problem is that of increased myocardial irritability due to acute myocardial infarction, arteriosclerotic coronary disease, Digitalis intoxication, or abnormal blood chemistries. As a general rule, we can say that a heart that fibrillates has the capacity to contract, and in most cases the pH of the blood at the moment of fibrillation is compatible with life. Therefore, the immediate effort should be directed to reversing the electrical changes by electric shock and on occasions by the use of Lidocaine or similar drugs. Most of the time, both procedures will be combined. But after the initial measures have been applied, determination of blood gases and pH is also important for two reasons:

a. The cardiac output may have stopped for a sufficiently long period of time as to produce some degree of lactic acidemia.

b. Previous abnormalities of the pH, oxygenation or ventilation may have been significant factors in producing the ventricular fibrillation.

If cardiac output is not restored promptly, serial determinations of blood gases are necessary, as often as every few minutes if possible, and ventilation, oxygenation and administration of bicarbonate adjusted according to the results obtained. We see in the literature at times the rule of blindly giving one ampule of bicarbonate for every five minutes of cardiac arrest. We think that this is very dangerous practice because if the lack of cardiac output is absolute, the administration of one ample of bicarbonate every five minutes will not change the outlook at all. On the other hand, if some cardiac output is being maintained through external massage, the use of one ampule of bicarbonate every five minutes is completely arbitrary and it may lead to values of pH too high or too low that would be incompatible with life. For guidelines on how much bicarbonate to give in a case of lactic acidemia following ventricular fibrillation, please see the chapter on therapy of metabolic acidemia.

3. When the heart stops as a result of *progressive bradycardia,* in cases where vital functions have been deteriorating progressively, one can be almost certain that at the time of death, the pH of the patient was very low. This would be due in some cases to metabolic acidemia and in others to hypoventilation. Most situations will have a combination of both. At which level of pH the heart stops would vary according to the general condition of the patient. A healthy young individual may still have a viable cardiac output when the pH is as low as 6.8 and an elderly patient with poor myocardium may go into asystole when the pH drops to values in the neighborhood of 7.1. The typical progression of changes in the electrocardiogram in such cases is as follows: With or without an in-between period of tachycardia, the regular sinus rhythm is followed by progressive bradycardia, which initially is of sinus origin and later on becomes nodal. The QRS complex starts widening and so does the T wave. The ST segment is usually somewhat elevated. As these changes and the bradycardia progress, the patient would, in most occasions, change to ventricular rhythm with wider and wider QRS complex and with smaller and smaller amplitude in the same. Ventricular fibrillation may or may not set in at any given point in this process of progressive deterioration. In most occasions, mechanical contraction of the heart will stop before the electrical complexes cease, giving way to a complete dissociation between mechanical and electrical activities of the heart. If the processes of acidemia, hypoxia and hypercapnea are reversed, in most instances the electrocardiographic changes will regress also following the opposite pattern than the one described. How viable the patient would be depends more than anything else on the damage suffered to the central nervous system.

These cases of cardiac arrests that follow progressive bradycardia and deterioration of vital functions are the ones that have greater possibility of being reversed or prevented. Careful observation of chronically ill patients and measurement of blood gases when clinically the situation seems to be deteriorating, may give us sufficient clues as to start the therapeutic measures that may prevent the cardiac arrest. The specific maneuvers to be undertaken to prevent the cardiac arrest would differ from patient to patient according to the nature of his basic problem and the degree of abnormality encountered in the measurements of his blood gases and pH. But, in general, adequate correction of abnormalities of pH, ventilation and oxygenation will be lifesaving until more basic therapy is insituted.

Awareness of the importance of taking preventive action in the situations described is what prompts some physicians to say that an intensive care unit where many dramatic cardiopulmonary resuscitation efforts are undertaken is probably not a very good unit, because with adequate preventive measures, some of these procedures may have never been needed. When a patient is fully controlled, all necessary measurements are being done and corrective action is being taken, and in spite of everything, the heart finally stops, the chances of success in active cardiopulmonary resuscitation are very small.

Once the cardiac arrest has occurred, the steps to be taken in the resuscitative effort are well standardized and it is not our purpose to repeat them again here in detail. We will just remind the reader of the great importance of keeping the airways open, ventilating the patient adequately, preferably with a high concentration of oxygen, correcting abnormalities of the acid-base balance and of the other chemicals of the blood that may have been a contributing factor to the arrest, and on occasions using skillfully some drugs that would enhance the contractivity of the myocardium or suppress its irritability. We want to warn against the excessive haste in intubating a patient in the midst of the resuscitative efforts in a case of cardiac arrest. The few seconds, or at times minutes, lost in an effort to intubate by a person who is poorly trained to do so, may be the difference between death and survival of the patient. Effective ventilation can be accomplished most of the times with an effective oropharyngeal airway, a tight mask and a ventilation bag. We resort to intubation only after we have obtained a viable cardiac output with a stable electrocardiographic pattern and we think that the patient can remain stable for twenty to thirty seconds without assisted ventilation. Also, we would like to emphasize that the use of drugs in cardiac arrest must be very judicious. One or two sympathomimetic drugs, one or two drugs to depress excessive irritability of the myocardium and adequate understanding of their pharmacological properties by the person in charge of the resuscitative effort will bring many more successes than the use of drug after drug in ever-increasing amounts without adequate judgement.

We are faced time and again with the question of when the resuscitative effort should be abandoned. There is no simple answer to this question. Previous condition of the patient, likelihood of reversibility of the events that led to the cardiac arrest, neurological status of the patient (pupils, reflexes, etc.) and many other factors are taken into consideration. In some occasions we have obtained some help in making such a decision from the study of peripheral arterial blood. Blood that has been stagnant in the artery for several minutes, as it would be in the case of a patient who still has some electrical activity but whose mechanical pumping action has stopped, follows a pattern of changes in the pH, pO_2, pCO_2 similar to what we would observe in blood that is maintained in a heparinized syringe at 37° Centigrade: the pO_2 decreases relatively fast as oxygen is being used by the blood cells, CO_2 increases as a result of cell metabolism and pH decreases accordingly. When there is no circulation at all, no lactic acid pours into the blood and the degree of acidemia is commensurate only to the degree of increase in the pCO_2. It is not unusual in some circumstances to obtain in the arterial blood values of pH around 7.20, pO_2 10-15 mm Hg, pCO_2 between 50 and 60 mm Hg. By contrast, if circulation is being maintained and ventilation is adequate by mechanical means with high concentration of oxygen, we would expect to have in the peripheral arterial blood a very good pO_2. If cardiac output is adequate, there would be little or no metabolic acidemia. If cardiac output is present but less than adequate, metabolic acidemia will result. In summary, only as a general guideline and without trying to make the rule absolute, values of peripheral blood in a case of cardiac arrest may indicate one of the following:

1. Stagnant blood: Moderately low pH, moderately high pCO_2, very low pO_2;

2. Circulation present with adequate cardiac output: Adequate values of pH, pO_2 and pCO_2;

3. Cardiac output present but insufficient: Good pO_2, good pCO_2, progressively decreasing pH.

REFERENCES

Camarath, S. J. et al.: Cardiac arrest in the critically ill. I. A study of predisposing causes in 132 patients. *Circulation, 44*:688, 1971.

Castagna, J. et al.: Factors determining survival in patients with cardiac arrest. *Chest, 65*:527, 1974.

El-Etr, A. A.: The management of cardiac arrest. *Surg. Clin., N. Amer, 48:* 17, 1968.

Goldberg, A. H.: Cardiopulmonary arrest. *New Eng. J. Med., 290*:381, 1974.

Harrison, D. C.: Acid-base changes during and following cardiac resuscitation. *Calif. Med., 118*:47, 1973.

Johnstone, R. E.: Cardiopulmonary resuscitation. *J.A.M.A., 228*:977, 1974.

Standards for cardiopulmonary resuscitation (CPR) and emergency cardiac care (ECC). *J.A.M.A., 227*:837, 1974.

CHAPTER IX

BLOOD GASES IN NEUROLOGICAL DISORDERS

CEREBROVASCULAR ACCIDENT

EVEN IF THE MAJORITY of patients with recent cerebrovascular accident may not manifest acute cardiorespiratory distress, a significant number, however, become acutely ill and in need of lifesaving therapeutic measures which are best provided in the intensive care setting. Several things occur in the acute CVA patient that contribute to create such critical situations:

1. Malfunction of the respiratory centers and of the cortex. Bilateral cortical involvement by direct lesion or by generalized edema of the brain may liberate the respiratory centers of the base of the brain from the moderating influence of the cortex, and as a result many of these patients with acute CVA would develop the so-called "central hyperventilation." In other occasions, the respiratory centers themselves are affected and marked hypoventilation may occur. Also, in some cases when the medulla is infarcted, even the most basic mechanisms of respiratory drive are affected and the patient may develop the so-called "Biot's respiration" with irregular pattern of breathing.

2. Increased production of bronchial secretions is often present (bronchorrhea) probably on a reflex basis.

3. The common mechanisms of defense of the glottic reflex and cough are significantly depressed.

4. Finally, in part, because of the fact that these patients are frequently old and, in part, because of the neurological damage of the CVA itself, normal mechanism of defense, such as turning in bed, taking occasional deep breaths, etc., are impaired. Also, because of the complete dependence of the patient on outside help, even for satisfaction of the water and electrolyte needs and because of the imperfect function of the kidneys and other vital or-

gans in elderly patients, it is very easy for these patients to develop electrolyte imbalance, hypoproteinemia, and other abnormalities that will affect the performance of the respiratory muscles.

Because of all the factors described, it is not uncommon to find the patients with a recent CVA in acute cardiorespiratory distress, cyanotic, with audible rhonchi and wheezes, appearing critically ill. A quick determination of arterial blood gases and pH can shed valuable light on the problem and may help in developing the guidelines of care.

I. The most common situation would be that of a patient with a moderate degree of hyperventilation, manifested by low pCO_2 and high pH, and at the same time having a moderate degree of hypoxia. In such a situation, the pulmonary difficulties are only minor, and we usually use oxygen by nasal cannula and a few treatments a day of mechanical ventilation with a face mask. General measures of adequate positioning of the patient, as well as attention to other medical problems, of course, should not be neglected.

2. Patients with a greater degree of unconsciousness and with more pulmonary involvement benefit at times from the introduction of an orotracheal tube, even when mechanical ventilation is not necessary. The presence of the tube would facilitate access to the bronchial secretions and endotracheal suction can be performed as often as needed. Also, oxygen could be applied in appropriate manner along with humidification by the use of a T tube connected to a nebulizer driven by a mixture of oxygen and air. Finally, if the clinical situation suddenly deteriorates, mechanical ventilation could be started at a moment's notice.

3. In cases of marked depression of the central nervous system with obvious hypoventilation, mechanical assistance will be necessary.

When ventilating patients with CVA mechanically, we should consider the particular situation of each patient and conduct mechanical ventilation accordingly. Some of these patients have basically little or no lung disease, their main problem being lack of respiratory drive. In such situations, we may be able to ventilate with very little pressure when using a pressure-controlled ventilator. Determination of tidal volumes and frequent measurement of arterial blood gases would be essential in adjusting the respirator.

We should also consider that in cases where the severe CVA is accompanied by hypothermia, the CO_2 production of the patient may be very small, at times no more than one-third of the usual, and ventilation has to be adjusted accordingly. Hyperventilation with a mechanical respirator is particularly dangerous in patients with central nervous diseases, because it is well known that hypocapnea is a powerful cerebral vasoconstrictor, and constriction of the cerebral arteries can further deprive the brain of oxygen, aggravating the intitial problem. In some of our patients with hypotherma, we have needed a little as 3 liters of minute ventilation in order to maintain adequate pH and pCO_2. When the cardiocirculatory system is involved and the patient goes into shock, in addition to all the appropriate measures to treat such a condition, administration of sodium bicarbonate may be necessary in order to compensate the progressive lactic acidosis. This therapy should be based on careful evaluation of the acid-base balance of the patient through repeated control of the arterial blood gases.

PSYCHOGENIC HYPERVENTILATION

It is not uncommon to see patients whose main complaints are "dizziness," "shortness of breath," and "fainting spells," without any obvious pulmonary impairment. When these problems occur in a young individual and no cardiopulmonary cause for the dyspnea is found, one has to think of the possibility of *psychogenic hyperventilation*. The chronology of a hyperventilation crisis is usually typical:

1. For no particular reason, but sometimes as a result of an unusual sensation inside the thorax, such as produced by paroxysmal atrial tachycardia or simple accumulation of mucus in the airways, the paient has a feeling of not having sufficient air in the lungs.

2. The patient then starts breathing fast and deep, sometimes as fast as fifty to sixty times per minute. After a few seconds, dizziness appears, perhaps accompanied by a sensation of numbness in fingers, arms or legs and, on occasions, also numbness around the mouth with a feeling of tingling in the lips and tongue.

3. Fainting or involuntary muscle contractions may follow, although this is not common. When they occur, these contractions

may be interpreted as an epileptic attack. However, they differ significantly from epilepsy in the sense that the patient most of the times would not lose consciousness completely, they are practically never accompanied by involuntary micturition, and the patient usually remembers what had happened before, during, and after the crisis.

The physiological changes behind this clinical picture are:

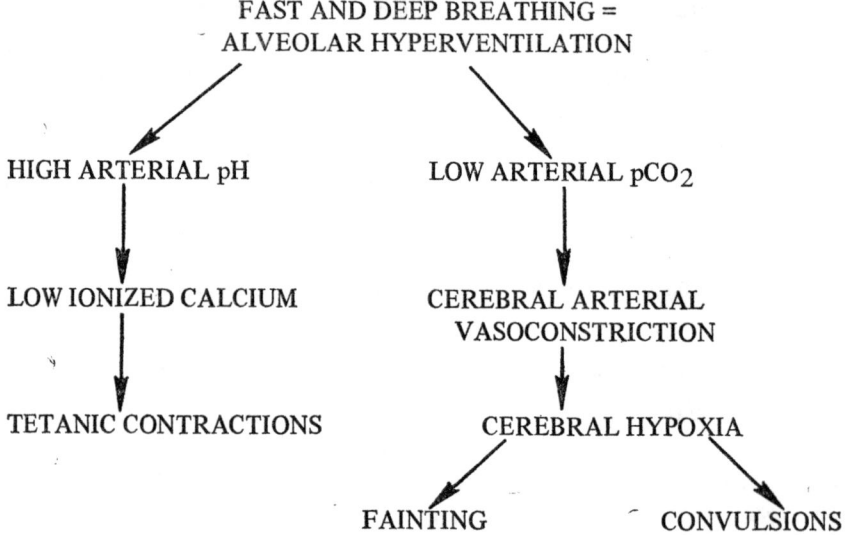

Even if not diagnostic, there are some characteristics that can be found in the pulmonary function tests and the arterial blood gases of the patients with psychogenic hyperventilation that may strongly support the diagnosis.

Blood gases usually would have a normal or high pH, normal or high pO_2, mildly or moderately low pCO_2 and mild or moderate deficit of plasma bicarbonate.

Example: pH 7.50, pO_2 100 mm Hg, pCO_2 25 mm Hg, bicarbonate 19.5 mEq/L.

These are patients who are usually very conscious of their own breathing and have a tendency to chronically hyperventilate. As a result, they maintain a slightly low pCO_2 at all times and with time, the bicarbonate is adjusted to those levels of pCO_2 in a way that the pH would remain within normal limits. During an acute hyperventilation crisis, the pCO_2 will decrease even more and a high pH will be obtained. Some degree of hyperventilation with acutely low pCO_2 and high pH is found many times, at the time of the arterial puncture, in patients who are otherwise stable. This type of hyperventilation as a reaction to the performance of the procedure, is quite common and should not be mistaken for the hyperventilation syndrome.

In performing the pulmonary function tests on these patients, normal function is usually found. However, when obtaining the functional residual capacity the tidal volume is recorded breath by breath for five to ten minutes, and we may find that these patients have a very irregular breathing pattern.

No standard approach to this problem can be developed that would fit all of the cases. Several points, however, may be of some benefit.

1. Correction of the initial abnormality that may trigger the hyperventilation crises such as control of paroxysmal atrial tachycardia when it exists, improvement of chronic bronchitis, etc.

2. Frank explanation of the problem to the patient. We have found very useful the approach of reproducing a near crisis by asking the patient to hyperventilate consciously and also showing the result of the pulmonary function test and blood gases and explaining the pathophysiology discussed above.

3. Some patients can be taught to control their pattern of breathing in a way that hyperventilation may be avoided. We have to emphasize in this respect the adoption of a slow respiratory rate. Some patients are able to achieve it by keeping their own respiratory rate to ten or eleven per minute while actually looking at their watch. Others may be able to slow the pattern of breathing by counting mentally to ten or fifteen during each expiration.

EPILEPTIC ATTACK

The pattern of blood gases observed immediately after a severe epileptic attack deserves particular attention. Even when the attack is triggered, as it is usually the case, by factors that have nothing to do with abnormalities of the acid-base balance, we may find after a severe prolonged epileptic attack a pattern of metabolic acidemia in the blood gases. We have seen cases where the bicarbonate concentration of the plasma immediate after the attack was no more than 7 or 8 mEq/liter and even with a moderate degree of compensatory hyperventilation, the pH was in the 7.1 range. The reason for these changes is usually the accumulation of lactic acid as a result of the increased muscular activity during the epileptic attack. We have to be careful not to make a diagnosis of metabolic derangement as a cause of the seizure when, in most instances, the abnormalities described are purely the results of the attack itself. Probably some of the so-called "metabolic encephalopathies" believed at times to be responsible for the convulsion never existed before the convulsion.

Unless the drop in the pH is extremely severe or the patient has other complications that may endanger his life, it is usually safe to leave these abnormalities of the acid-base balance metabolism untreated because the lactic acid most likely will be metabolized back into bicarbonate and homeostasis will be again achieved. Overreacting to the situation and replacing the lost plasma bicarbonate would bring a moderate degree of metabolic alkalemia later on once the circulating lactic acid has been metabolized. Blood gases taken two hours after the convulsions are usually normal again. We must not forget, however, that convulsions can really occur as a result of the abnormalities of the electrolytes and acid-base balance. The severe hypoxia that occurs as a result of mraked cerebral vasconstriction resulting from hyperventilation can be a cause of convulsions. Also, marked hyponatremia and other abnormalities of the electrolyte picture, as well as severe acidemia, may trigger an epileptic attack in some patients.

ARTERIOSCLEROSIS OF THE CEREBROVASCULAR SYSTEM

As the blood vessels of the brain and the cerebral function deteriorate, even without clear cerebrovascular accident, many patients develop one of the following abnormalities in their pattern of breathing:

1. *Central hyperventilation.* This is a very common feature.

Senile patients, particularly if they are somewhat confused, very commonly hyperventilate in a chronic manner. It is not uncommon in these patients to have a minimally elevated pH with a moderately low pCO_2 and a moderately low plasma bicarbonate. The following figures would represent a typical example:

pH 7.475, pO_2 70 mm Hg, pCO_2 28 mm Hg, bicarbonate 20.5 mEq/L.

Fortunately, hyperventilation in patients with advanced arteriosclerotic vascular disease of the brain appears not to be as harmful as it would be in younger individuals. It has been demonstrated experimentally that the decrease in blood flow to the brain of an arteriosclerotic patient, as a result of hyperventilation, is much less than in younger individuals who have the capability of constricting the arteries. In the senile patient, apparently, the arteries are more or less fixed and hyperventilation produces little vasoconstriction. No specific therapy appears to be effective in such a situation and probably none is needed. We use some oxygen, however, when this hyperventilation is accompanied by hypoxia or by signs of significant distress.

2. Senile patients, because of progressive dysfunction of the cortex, revert many times to *Cheyne-Stokes* pattern of breathing. This is particularly well noticed during sleep, but occurs also in patients who are conscious, but slightly confused. We have not found this to be particularly harmful. We use oxygen in such cases when the general condition warrants it.

OVERDOSE

Patients with overdose of barbituates or related substances may develop acute respiratory failure and may be in need of assisted mechanical ventilation. The problem becomes at times more complicated because some of the drugs commonly involved in overdose cases may produce convulsions. As a result, these patients often receive barbituates for the treatment of the convulsions, compounding the problem of depression of the respiratory center. When respiratory failure is diagnosed on clinical and laboratory grounds (blood gases), intubation and mechanical ventilation are indicated. In general, these patients tolerate the endotracheal tube very well because if they are in need of mechanical ventilation, their reflexes are usually depressed enough that the presence of the endotracheal tube may not produce much reaction on the part of the patient. Because these patients may vomit and aspirate, and because some of the drugs involved may have a delayed action, we at times intubate a patient even with normal blood gases if we see clinical signs of a marked depression of reflexes and the patient is completely unconscious. With adequate support of ventilation and with judicious medical management, most patients with overdose who arrive alive at the hospital will survive. Death from respiratory depression is practically always preventable if the patient is taken to the hospital in time. On occasions, even with adequate mechanical ventilation, death may still occur due to cardiovascular shock, renal failure or other complications.

In general, tracheostomy is very seldom needed in cases of overdose because the endotracheal tube is usually well tolerated and the period of time when mechanical assistance is needed very few times extends to more than a few days.

REFERENCES

Currier, R. D. et al.: Acute cerebral infarction—evaluation and treatment. *Postgrad. Med., 54*:83, 1973.

Greer, M.: Management of the patient with acute stroke. *Geriatr., 28*:48, 1973.

Hill, P. M.: Hyperventilation, breath holding and alveolar oxygen tensions at the breaking point. *Resp. Physiol., 19*:201, 1973.

Murrin, K. R. et al.: Hyperventilation and psychometric testing. A preliminary study. *Anaesthesia, 29*:50, 1974.

Simand, D. et al.: Artificial hyperventilation in stroke. *Trans. Am. Neurol. Assoc., 98*:309, 1973.

CHAPTER X

BLOOD GASES IN NEUROMUSCULAR DISORDERS

THE GUILLAIN-BARRE SYNDROME

THIS DISEASE IS USUALLY a reversible polyneuritis that in most instances of moderately severe intensity will affect the muscles of respiration and induce respiratory failure.

Most of these patients will need ventilatory support. In children with only moderate involvement, we have found successful at times the technique of helping them with the tank respirator without having to do a tracheostomy. This is usually possible when the patient is conserving some respiratory muscle capability and his main problem is fatigue. By using the tank he can be supported in his ventilation most of the time, but yet, he would be able to ventilate on his own for short periods of time when opening the tank or when adjusting controls. In cases of very severe respiratory paralysis where the patient is unable to ventilate on his own at all, tracheostomy is mandatory and mechanical ventilation is applied as needed in a supportive manner. We have to be mindful of the fact that, in general, these patients have healthy lungs and that ventilation with room air or with slightly increased concentration of oxygen, is preferable to high oxygen concentrations.

In the adult patients, particularly if they are relatively obese, the tank respirator is usually not effective and we have to do tracheostomy and to support ventilation mechanically. These patients have a great tendency to develop respiratory infections and the problem of the respiratory failure may be complicated with parenchymatous lung disease. These patients need not only mechanical support, but very careful observation and judicious therapy of all possible complicating factors. For more details, please see the chapter on mechanical ventilation.

POLIOMYELITIS

We have not seen cases of active poliomyelitis in years. The problem has been well studied in the past and if a new case is to be treated, we would refer the reader to the pertinent literature. What we still see now very frequently are the complications of previous polio in patients who have been left with diminished respiratory reserve. Most of the patients that we followed are relatively stable. Some of them have had corrective surgery. They are in a borderline status in their respiratory function and the main problems are usually acute episodes of decompensation when complications occur. The most common complications that we have seen in recent years resulting in acute decompensation have been pregnancy, pulmonary tuberculosis and acute bacterial or viral pulmonary infections. It is significant that most patients with chronic polio and marked degree of pulmonary function impairment usually maintain good oxygenation of the blood, provided that they can ventilate adequately and that they are relatively young. However, as age advances, even if ventilation is maintained adequately, they in time develop hypoxia because of the progressive deterioration of the lung tissue itself and the result of repeated pulmonary infections. In this sense, they behave very much as the kyphoscoliotic patients do. As time goes on and these patients develop hypoxia, cor pulmonale is a very real danger.

Treatment in these cases will depend very much on the individual situation. In young individuals who develop acute respiratory failure, we have had success by using the tank respirator during the time that the acute complication was present. Most of these patients are used to this type of therapy and they adjust very well, since many of them used it as children during their acute period of disease.

MYASTHENIA GRAVIS

Patients with severe myasthenia gravis often develop acute respiratory failure. The two most common causes of respiratory failure are:

1. Deterioration of the disease per se, with increased muscle weakness and,

2. Pulmonary complications, such as bronchopneumonia that would make ventilation more difficult, even if the muscle strength has not been decreased.

When the problem is only increasing weakness without parenchymatous pulmonary complication, usually these patients are only mildly hypoxic. However, when the problem is pulmonary infection, the patients usually develop marked hypoxia. In the acute phase of decompensation with hypoxia and CO_2 retention, we have found very successful the technique of intubation and mechanical ventilation. Usually, these patients tolerate the tube relatively well and in a few days the pulmonary problem can be solved and the ventilatory capability of the patient returns to acceptable levels. Usually no more than three or four days of mechanical ventilation have been required in most of the cases that we have treated. We prefer to avoid tracheostomy in these cases if possible because usually the disease is self-limited and in a few days these patients can do well without having to face the possible complications of the tracheostomy and the longer recovery period that inevitably follows.

In patients who, in addition to myastenia gravis, have some degree of arteriosclerotic cardiovascular disease and chronic obstructive pulmonary disease, usually the situation is very difficult to handle. These patients require increased muscle strength to ventilate because of their chronic obstructive lung disease and they are more apt to develop acute respiratory failure. Also, we are somewhat limited in the use of drugs, if they have significant arterioscleriotic cardiovascular disease. Some of the drugs used in the treatment of the myasthenia itself would have an ionotropic effect on the heart and would favor the production of arrhythmia in someone who already has arteriosclerotic cardiovascular problems. Also, the medication that is required to treat bronchospasm can induce cardiac arrhythmia. The treatment of these patients becomes very complicated and quite often is not very successful. Due to the limitiations in the use of the drugs, we have found ourselves having to be more aggressive in the use of mechanical ventilation for prolonged periods of time. Tracheostomy is necessary when mechanical ventilation is contemplated for more than five or six days. The combination of advanced age, myasternia, chronic obstructive disease of the lungs and arteriosclerotic cardiovascular disease is a very difficult one and the prognosis of the patient, most of the times, is very poor.

AMYOTROPHIC LATERAL SCLEROSIS

Many patients with amyotrophic lateral sclerosis eventually succumb to respiratory failure. This is particularly true when the process combines with chronic obstructive disease of the lungs. The usual course of events is the development of respiratory failure when a superimposed respiratory infection increases the work of breathing in these patients. They usually need mechanical ventilation, and they usually need it for a long time, requiring tracheostomy and continued ventilatory support. Many patients will recover from the first episode of acute respiratory failure, but as the neuromuscular and respiratory processes progress, the patients invariably find themselves again in acute respiratory failure and the recovery becomes every time more difficult.

TETANUS

Since the advent of mechanical ventilation, many cases of tetanus have been saved. These patients are usually managed with tracheostomy, curarization and mechanical ventilation. Of course, many more things are needed, such as the use of antitetanus globulin, antibiotics, and judicious use of general supportive medication. From the respiratory point of view, we should be prepared for a prolonged struggle of several weeks of mechanical ventilation in a patient who is almost totally dependent on the ventilator, almost completely paralyzed by the use of curare type drugs. In spite of the best care, some patients will die of toxic myocarditis.

REFERENCES

Brown, W. F. et al.: Amyotrophic lateral sclerosis. Electrophysiologic study. *Arch. Neurol.*, *30*:242, 1974.
Engel, W. K. et al.: Myasthenia gravis. *Am. Intern. Med.*, *81*:225, 1974.
Selecry, P. A. et al.: Prolonged respirator support for the treatment of intractable myasthenia gravis. *Chest*, *65*, 1974.

CHAPTER XI

BLOOD GASES IN THE RESPIRATORY DISTRESS SYNDROME OF THE ADULT

RESPIRATORY DISTRESS SYNDROME OF THE ADULT (RDSA)

THIS IS A DEVASTATING CONDITION that can occur in a variety of situations. Biochemically, it is characterized by a marked decrease in the amount of "surfactant" in the lung tissue, this in turn, producing a greater tendency toward exudation of fluids in the interstitial spaces of the lung and to production of diffuse generalized microatelectases. Physiologically, we find the lung tissue to be very stiff, the work of breathing markedly increased, the physiological dead space also greatly increased and the transfer of oxygen significantly impaired. Clinically, these patients appear severely hypoxic, often mentally confused and disoriented, always with great respiratory distress if they are not assisted mechanically in their ventilation.

Many names have been given to this syndrome: Da-Nang lung (because it was observed very frequently and studied during the Vietnam War), shock lung, "respirator lung," etc. It can occur as a result of chest trauma, severe generalized infections, severe hypotension, prolonged use of mechanical ventilation, especially if high concentrations of oxygen are used, and a variety of other medical conditions characterized by their severity. Particularly difficult to treat has been the respiratory distress syndrome that we have encountered in cases of pneumocystis carinii pneumonia in patients on immunosuppressive drugs.

On physiological and clinical grounds we may have a strong suspicion of dealing with a case of respiratory distress syndrome of the adult when the two following conditions are present:

1. Hazy, diffuse infiltration of the entire lung field;

2. Marked hypoxia even when using high concentrations of oxygen.

The patients with RDSA invariably need mechanical ventilation. Since they will need it for prolonged periods of time, a tracheostomy becomes necessary, even if an endotracheal tube could have been placed initially to solve the emergency situation.

When ventilating patients with RDSA, the following points should be considered:

1. PEEP (Positive End Expiratory Pressure) should be used. In general, we use 8 to 10 cm of PEEP. By keeping some positive pressure inside the lungs at all times during the respiratory cycle, the alveolar units of the lungs are more apt to remain open and oxygenation is significantly improved. It is not uncommon to see patients with RDSA who are on a ventilator without the PEEP and who may have a paO_2 of no more than 40 mm Hg even with an F_IO_2 of 0.7 or 0.8, and the paO_2 will increase to as much as 60 mm Hg when the PEEP is applied, without changing the F_IO_2.

2. High inspiratory flows are usually required because most of these patients do not have airway obstruction and they have a tendency to breathe forcefully, in part due to the sensation of air hunger that the syndrome produces. In young adults, flows of 80 to 100 liters per minute are used.

3. The physiological dead space of these patients is greatly increased as a result of the changes in the lung parenchyma. Even with the mechanical assistance, the work of breathing is increased unless they are paralyzed pharmacologically. Because of all these factors, large tidal volumes and large minute ventilations are necessary. In some cases we have used values as high as 1,000 cc of tidal volume and respiratory rate of twenty-five to thirty per minute in order to obtain normal arterial pCO_2. It is quite rewarding to see that as the disease improves and the lungs clear, smaller and smaller minute ventilations are needed.

4. The F_IO_2 has to be adjusted very carefully. On one hand, due to the very severe hypoxia of these patients, very high concentrations of oxygen in the inspired air may be necessary. On the other hand, the higher the concentration of oxygen used, the more damage to the lung tissue will occur, aggravating the RDSA itself and precipitating at times a vicious circle of

hypoxia → higher F_IO_2 → more damage to the lung tissues → more hypoxia.

Because of all these considerations, we try to use the lowest F_IO_2 possible that would still give us a relatively comfortable paO_2. As a general rule we are satisfied with paO_2 of 50 mm Hg and we do not try to obtain higher values if, in order to do so, we had to use F_IO_2 above 0.4 or 0.45. Since the conditions that affect oxygenation and ventilation can change very rapidly in patients with severe RDSA, we obtain arterial blood gases in these patients at least every twelve hours.

5. The feeling of "air hunger" in these patients is such that in many occasions they try to override the respiratory rate of the mechanical ventilator and trigger the machine at a faster rate producing some degree of hyperventilation and respiratory alkalemia. Most of the times this is not detrimental to the patient and no corrective action is necessary provided that the problem does not become extreme. In very extreme situations we may have to curarize the patient in order to control ventilation adequately. When using curare or similar drugs we should be careful of giving the smallest dosage that would allow us to obtain our objectives of adequate ventilation without completely paralyzing the patient if possible. A patient who is able to ventilate spontaneously, even if with difficulty and for short periods of time, is much safer on the ventilator than a completely paralyzed patient because the possibility of disconnection of the machine or malfunction of the same is always present.

6. We have to realize that usually mechanical ventilation will be continued for several weeks, on occasions as much as two months. Therefore, we should be careful in organizing everything that pertains to the care of the patient for such prolonged periods of mechanical assistance. We have found of very great importance the following points.

    a. It is very easy to produce erosion of the tracheal wall with at times catastrophic results when mechanical ventilation has to be prolonged for more than eight to ten days. Tracheal esophageal fistula may develop. Erosion into a large blood vessel is always a possibility. Even if none of these occur, endotracheal strictures may appear at a later date. Because of all these factors, extreme care has to be taken with the positioning of the tracheostomy tube and with the care of the balloon. We have found that at times we can obtain good results by having a relatively high tracheostomy and using a longer tracheostomy tube with two balloons that can be inflated alternately. Alternating inflation of the balloons will decrease the danger of erosion at any given point; a greater length of tracheostomy tube in the trachea will keep the tube in a more stable position in the midline and avoid to some extent the scratching of the tracheal wall by the tip of the tube. As little air as possible should be introduced in the balloons. The amount of air introduced should not be always constant but should be determined at the time of its inflation. In general, we like to start the respirator first and then to slowly add air to the balloon until we find the machine working properly, preferably leaving a small leak between the cuff and the tracheal wall.

    b. Suction should be done carefully and very briefly. It is extremely important not to suction the patient for more than 4 or 5 seconds at a time. Cardiac arrest due to extreme hypoxia is a great danger in these patients when endotracheal suction is unduly prolonged. In very severe cases it may be wise to ventilate the patient with 100% oxygen for three or four minutes before suctioning. If more than three or four seconds is necessary for suction, we should stop it at the end of this period of time, put the patient back on the respirator for a few breaths and then resume suction again for very short periods of time.

    c. Marked hypoalbuminemia is encountered very frequently in these patients. This may be in part due to the fact that nutrition of a patient on the respirator at times may be neglected when everyone is preoccupied by keeping the lungs going. In many cases, however, there appears to be a very rapid turnover of albumin and even with good nutrition hypoalbuminemia can develop. This is particularly striking in cases of RDSA secondary to pneumocystis carinii pneumonia in patients on immunosuppressive drugs. We have found it necessary at times to determine the levels of albumin and proteins every day and to replace the albumin intravenously on a daily basis.

It appears that as long as the serum albumin is very low, the lung problems are much more difficult to correct, probably in part due to the fact that low oncotic pressures favor the production of interstitial pneumonic infiltration. We like to keep the albumin of these patients above 3 gm/100 cc.

    d. Good electrolyte balance is necessary and most of the time daily determination of electrolytes may be required in order to correct possible abnormalities. In general, it is much easier to maintain normal electrolytes if we place a nasogastric tube as soon as mechanical ventilation is initiated and feed and hydrate the patient adequately through the nasogastric tube.

    e. These patients are extremely susceptible to develop tracheal and pulmonary infections. Careful sterile techniques should be used by all personnel that would enter the room of the patient. They should be maintained practically in the socalled "reverse isolation." They should be protected adequately with antibiotics. Frequent cultures of tracheal secretions should be done.

The process of weaning of RDSA patients from the respirator is at times a protracted one. No definite guidelines can be given because we will have to act in every case according to the particular situation. In general, we try to decrease the PEEP when we see that we can obtain adequate oxygenation with concentrations of oxygen of 35% or lower. If the situation remains stable after PEEP is discontinued and the minute ventilation required to maintain adequate arterial pCO_2 has decreased to reasonable levels, usually 10 liters per minute or less, we may try to allow the patient to have progressive periods of spontaneuos ventilation.

    f. Throughout the entire period of mechanical ventilation we must be aware of the fact that pneumothorax is a very frequent complication and may require prompt action on the part of the respiratory team.

REFERENCES

Acute pulmonary injury and repair (the adult respiratory distress syndrome). The 16th Aspen Lung Conference. *Chest, 65,* April 1974, Supplement. Edited by T. L. Petty and L. D. Hudson.

Blaisdell, F. W.: Pathophysiology of the respiratory distress syndrome. *Arch. Surg., 108:*44, 1974.

Bredenberg, S. E.: Acute respiratory distress. *Surg. Clin. N. Amer., 54:*1043, 1974.

King, T. K. et al.: Oxygen transfer in catastrophic respiratory failure. *Chest, 65,* Supplement 40S-44S, 1974.

Petty, T. L., and Ashbaugh, D. G.: The respiratory distress syndrome. *Chest, 60*:233, 1971.

Sutton, F. D.: Recognition and management of the adult respiratory distress syndrome. *Chest, 66,* Supplement 34S-36S, 1974.

CHAPTER XII

BLOOD GASES IN MISCELLANEOUS PROBLEMS

CHEST WALL PROBLEMS

1. Kyphoscoliosis.

KYPHOSCOLIOSIS, BY DEFORMING the thoracic cage and altering the mechanics of the lung, can lead to severe pulmonary failure and cor pulmonale. When testing the lung function of a kyphoscoliotic child, the following results are usually obtained.

a. *Lung volumes.* Residual volume is many times close to normal. Total lung capacity is decreased and the ratio between residual volume and total lung capacity is increased. The decrease in thoracic volume tends to decrease the residual volume, and the rigidity of the thoracic wall tends to increase it, the result being a value very close to the predicted normal.

b. *Ventilatory studies.* There is usually no obstruction of the airways in the early stages of the disease. The ventilatory studies expressed as percentage of the predicted values is usually as good, or even better, than the same value of lung volumes.

c. *Distribution studies.* Distribution of inspired air is minimally altered and the nitrogen washout will be very close to normal.

d. *Diffusion studies.* Carbon monoxide diffusing capacity is decreased by a percentage usually in proportion to the decrease of lung volumes, indicating a normal transfer of gases across the alveolar capillary barrier.

e. *Blood gases.* Most of these patients will usually have a normal pH and normal pO_2. The pCO_2 is sometimes slightly low due to the fact that the thoracic deformity brings on a conscious pattern of breathing and a chronic state of hyperventilation.

But as the age of the patient advances, the impaired mechanics of the lung make him more susceptible to pulmonary infections, leading to progressive destruction of the lung tissue, chronic bronchitis and hypoxia. The hypoxia in turn leads to sustained pulmonary hypertension, and cor pulmonale develops. It is not uncommon, as a result, to have middle age kyphoscoliotics with severe hypoxia, airway obstruction, cor pulmonale and eventual hypoventilation.

Because of this unfavorable progression of the disease, early correction of the kyphoscoliosis appears to be very important.

In order to evaluate the surgical risks and to outline the postoperative management of the pulmonary problems of these patients, a complete preoperative evaluation of the lung function and repeated postoperative blood gases will be very helpful. Patients who have normal blood gases before surgery, even in the presence of a moderate decrease of lung volumes, usually have a good postoperative prognosis. If the patient goes into acute respiratory failure after surgery, judicious use of the tank respirator with proper control of minute ventilation and blood gases can usually tide the patient over the first postoperative week and solve the problems. If blood gases were frankly abnormal before surgery, indicating the existence of marked hypoxia, the patient already has significant parenchymatous disease and probably cor pulmonale. In these cases, the postoperative course is much more difficult and usually tracheostomy with assisted mechanical ventilation will be necessary.

2. Flail Chest.

Patients with multiple rib fractures may develop paradoxical movements of the chest wall with respiration, consisting mainly in the depression during inspiration of the unsupported part of the chest wall. As a result, the inspiratory effort, even if increased, is many times insufficient to produce adequate alveolar ventilation. In addition, it is not uncommon to have serious damage to the lung parenchyma with the trauma and/or traumatic pneumothorax.

These patients would be very dyspneic and when determining the blood gases we would find a moderate degree of hypoxia with or without pCO_2 retention and acidemia.

In general, these patients need mechanical ventilation in order to support the function of the lungs and also to allow better mechanical conditions for stabilization and healing of the traumatized chest wall.

Even if endotracheal intubation can solve an emergency situation, usually most patients will require tracheostomy in order to receive mechanical ventilation for a few days or weeks. In ventilating these patients the following points are taken into consideration.

a. A few cm of PEEP will be very helpful in maintaining the chest slightly inflated, allowing for better stabilization of the chest wall and preventing trauma to the lung tissue by the broken ribs.

b. Relatively large inspiratory flow should be used in order to prevent the "sucking" of air by the patient, which would create a negative pressure inside the lungs, defeating the purpose of the PEEP. Since most of these patients have otherwise healthy lungs without airway obstruction, able to accept large inspiratory flows, it is not unusual to have to use flows as high as 80 to 100 liters per minute.

c. The concentration of oxygen in the inspired air will have to be adjusted according to the particular situation of the patient. In general, unless the trauma to the lung is very extensive, relatively low concentrations of oxygen in the range of 25 to 30% will be sufficent. Particular care has to be taken not to give higher concentrations of oxygen than absolutely necessary because the already damaged lung may be more susceptible to oxygen toxicity.

d. In the weaning process we first discontinue the PEEP while continuing the mechanical ventilation. If the chest remains stable and the clinical conditions favorable, the following day we may start the process of allowing the patient to breathe spontaneously at short intervals of time without assisted mechanical ventilation. Once this is accomplished without much distress to the patient, it is usually possible to discontinue all mechanical assistance in one to two more days.

DROWNING AND NEAR DROWNING

Victims of drowning and near drowning need intensive respiratory care. An excellent monograph on the subject has been published by Jerome H. Modell, M.D., in 1971 (see references at the end of this chapter). Because of our limited experience in treating victims of near drowning we would like to refer the reader to the above mentioned monograph.

REFERENCES

Block, A. M. et. al.: Cardiopulmonary failure of the hunchback. A possible therapeutic approach. *J.A.M.A., 212*:1520, 1970.

Fine, N. L. et. al.: Near drowning presenting as the adult respiratory distress syndrome. *Chest, 65*:347, 1974.

James, O. et. al.: Chest injury: The indications for artificial ventilation. *Anaesth. Intensive Care, 2*:27, 1974.

Lin, H. Y. et. al.: The effect of corrective surgery on pulmonary function in scoliosis. *J. Bone Joint Surg., 56A*:1173, 1974.

Modell, J. H.: *Drowning and Near-Drowning.* Springfield, Illinois: Thomas, 1971.

Rutledge, R. R. et. al.: The use of mechanical ventilation with positive-end-expiratory pressure in the treatment of near-drowning. *Anesthesiology, 38*:194, 1973.

Sladen, A. et. al.: PEEP & ZEEP in the treatment of flail chest injuries. *Crit. Care Med., 1*:187, 1973.

Webb, W. R.: Thoracic trauma. *Surg. Clin. N. Amer., 54*:1179, 1974.

Webb, W. R.: Flail chest. *Surg. Clin. N. Amer., 54*:1182, 1974.

Workman, J. M.: Lung disease in kyphoscoliosis. *Lancet, 2*:271, 1973.

Youmans, C. R. Jr. et. al.: Recognition and management of flail chest. *Med. Trial Tech. Quart., 20*:141, Fall 1973.

AUTHOR INDEX

A
Aberman, A., 81
Andrews, J.L., Jr., 36, 49
Ashbaugh, D.G., 106
Avery, W.G., 81
Ayres, S.M., 81

B
Barach, A.L., 63
Bartels, H., 13, 36
Bates, D.V., 36
Benediten, H.H., 75
Bergman, N.A., 63
Blaisdell, F.W., 105
Block, A.M., 110
Brackett, N.C., 49
Bredenberg, S.E., 105
Brown, W.F., 100

C
Camarath, S.J., 88
Campbell, E.J.M., 49
Castagna, J., 88
Chaves, A.D., 63
Christie, R.V., 36
Chusid, E.L., 75
Comroe, J., 13, 36, 42
Conference on the Scientific Basis of Respiratory Therapy, 49, 63
Crews, E.R., 36
Currier, R.D., 96

D
Degre, S., 63

E
El-Etr, A.A., 88
Engel, W.K., 100

F
Fenn, W.O., 13, 36
Filley, G.F., 13, 36
Fine, N.L., 110
Franklin, W., 75
Fulop, M, 81

G
Garella, S., 49
Goldberg, A.H., 88
Greer, M., 96
Gruzman, A.B., 75

H
Harrison, D.C., 88
Hill, P.M., 96

I
Ingram, R.H., 42

J
James, O., 110
Johnstone, R.E., 88

K
Karpick, R.J., 63
Kassirer, J.P., 49
King, T.K., 106

L
Laenec, R.T.H., 81
Lapuerta, L., 36
Lee, J., 36
Lin, H.Y., 110

Mc
Mc Mahon, S. M., 75

M
Meyer, J.A., 75
Miller, A., 81
Miller, W.F., 81
Modell, J.H., 110
Murrin, K.R., 96

N
Nadel, J.A., 63

P
Petty, L.T., 37
Petty, T.L., 63, 106
Powers, S.R., 75

R
Rahn, H., 13, 36
Rector, F.C., Jr., 37
Rutledge, R.R., 110

S
Schwartz, W.B., 37
Seldin, D.W., 37
Selecry, P.A., 100
Shapiro, B.A., 37
Simand, D., 96
Sladen, A., 110

Sproule, B.J., 81
Staub, N.C., 81
Sutton, F.D., 106
Symposium on Chronic Respiratory Disease, 63

T
Tierney, D.F., 63

W
Waltemath, C.L., 63
Webb, H.H., 63
Webb, W.R., 10
Workman, J.M., 110

Y
Youmans, C.R., Jr., 110

Z
Zwillich, C.W., 75

SUBJECT INDEX

A

Acetylsalycilic acid, 45 *(see also* Aspirin)
Acid-base balance, 16, 22-24, 27, 30, 31, 35, 45-49, 86, 93
   problems, 45-49
Acidemia, viii, 22, 24, 38-39, 46, 48, 49, 50, 82, 84, 108
   diabetic, 49
   lactic, 49, 79, 82, 84
   metabolic, 24-25, 29, 79, 85, 87
   renal, 49
   respiratory, 24, 38, 59, 76
Acidosis, 21
   diabetic, 30
   lactic, 39, 91
   metabolic, 23, 76
   respiratory, 23
      compensated, 27
Albumin, plasma, 73, 74, 104, 105
Alkalemia, 22, 24, 28, 35, 40-41, 47-48, 49, 67, 94
   metabolic, 25
   respiratory, 25, 103
Alkalosis
   "hypochloremic," 27
   metabolic, 23
   respiratory, 23
Alveoli, 7, 15, 17
   air, 6, 16
      carbon dioxide, *see* $PACO_2$
      nitrogen, *see* PAN_2
      oxygen, *see* PAO_2
   ventilation, 17, 22, 25, 28, 40
Anaerobiosis, 27, 39
Anemia, 10
Arrhythmia, cardiac, 56, 82, 83, 99
Arterial blood, 7
   carbon dioxide, *see* $paCO_2$
   gas measurement norms, 11
   nitrogen, *see* paN_2
   oxygen, *see* paO_2
Arteriosclerosis, 84, 94-95, 99
   cerebral, 29, 40
Aspirin encephalopathy, 46
Aspirin poisoning, 30, 45
Asthma, bronchial, 53
   treatment, 58-59
Asystole, sudden, 83-84
Atelectasis, pulmonary, 69, 70, 75
Atropine, 83

B

Base excess, 31
Barbituate overdose, 95-96
Bicarbonate, plasma *(see* Plasma bicarbonate)
Bilirubin, 39
Biot's respiration, 89
Blood
   acidity, 10-13
   arterial, *see* Arterial blood
   capillary, *see* Capillary blood
   gas transportation, 7-10
   ionic balance, 35
Brachial artery, 20
Bradycardia, 70, 83
   progressive, 85-88
Bronchitis, chronic, 51-52, 54, 55 93, 108
   IPPB treatments, 55-56
   oxygen, use of, 56-57
Bronchodilators, 38, 47, 55, 58
Bronchopneumonia, 99
Bronchorrhea, 89
Bronchospasm, 47, 51, 53, 54, 59, 65, 99

C

Calcium, viii, 35, 41
Capillary blood 6, 7, 16
   carbon dioxide, *see* $p\bar{c}CO_2$
   nitrogen, *see* $p\bar{c}N_2$
   oxygen, *see* $p\bar{c}O_2$

Carbon dioxide (CO_2), vii, 4, 5, 6, 7, 14, 15, 17, 28, 31, 50, 51, 87, 91, 107
  alveolar air, in, see $PACO_2$
  arterial blood, in, see $paCO_2$
  capillary blood, in see $p\bar{c}CO_2$
  elimination, 16-17
  inspired air, in, see $PICO_2$
  retention, 30, 38, 57, 60, 76, 99
  solubility coefficient, 6
  venous blood, mixed, in, see $p\bar{v}CO_2$
Cardiovascular shock, 29
Carbon monoxide, 8, 9
  intoxication, 32
Carbonic acid (H_2CO_3), 12
Cardiac arrest, 21, 82-88
Cardiopathies, congenital, 19
Cardiovascular shock, 29
Cardiovascular system, vii
Catacholamines, 47
Central nervous system, vii, 15
Cerebral edema, 38
Cerebrovascular accident, 29, 82, 89-91
Cheyne-Stokes breathing pattern, 95
Chlorides, 30, 35, 36, 41, 48
Cor pulmonale, 51, 52, 57, 98, 107, 108
Cromolyn sodium, 58
Curare, 103
Curarization, 100
Cyanosis, 39, 70, 76, 77

D

Da-Nang lung, 101
Dead space, physiological, 16, 17, 18, 28, 66, 101, 102
Dehydration, 82
Diffusion, gas, 3-5
  defect, 19
Digitalis, viii, 77, 78, 79, 80
  intoxication, 82
Diuretics, 30, 35, 48, 78, 79
Drowning, 76, 82, 109-110
Dyspnea, 40, 53, 91, 108

E

Edema
  cerebral, 38
  laryngeal, 71
  pulmonary, 19, 27, 56, 76-81

Electrode, blood gas, ix
Electrolytes, vii, viii, ix, 14, 15, 31, 34, 36, 38, 40, 94
  balance, 14, 34, 105
  derangement, 48
  disturbances, 81
  imbalance, 51, 79, 90
Emphysema, pulmonary, 52-53
  treatment, 57-58
Encephalopathies, metabolic, 94
Endotracheal tube, 44
Enzymes, vii, 8
Epilepsy, 92-94

F

Femoral artery, 20
Fibrillation, ventricular, 82, 83, 84
Flail chest 108-109
Furosemide 79, 80

G

Gas
  diffusion, 3-5
  mass movement, 3-5
  water solution, 5-7
Gas analysis
  arterial collection, 20-22
Gastrointestinal system, vii, viii
Glomeruli, 30
Glucose, vii
Guillain-Barre syndrome, 97

H

Hallucination, 39
Hematoma, 20
Hemodialysis, viii
Hemoglobin, 7, 8, 9, 22, 31, 32, 33, 38,
  dissociation curve, 32
  poisoning, 10
Hemorrhage, 82
Henderson-Hasselbalch equation, 12, 23, 25, 36
Heparin, 20
Hydrogen ions, vii, viii, 10, 11, 12, 13, 14, 15, 16, 24, 30
Hyperaldosteronism, 48
Hyperbasemia, 22-23, 28
Hypercalcemia, 82, 83
Hypercapnea, 22, 38, 50, 59, 78, 82, 85

Hyperoxygenation, 41-42
Hyperpotassemia, 34, 38, 82, 83
Hypertension, 39
  pulmonary, 51, 52, 57, 108
Hyperventilation, 28, 29, 40, 46, 47, 48, 90, 91 103, 107
  central, 89, 94
  psychogenic, 29, 91-93
Hypoalbuminemia, 104
Hypobasemia, 22-23, 45
Hypocapnea, 22, 40, 91
Hyponatremia, 34, 94
Hypopotassemia, 34, 40, 81
Hypoproteinemia, 90
Hypotension, 38, 39, 101
Hypothermia, 91
Hypothyroidism, 51
Hypoventilation, 28, 32, 43, 76, 78, 81, 82, 85, 89, 90, 108
Hypoxemia, arterial, 19-20
Hypoxia, tissue, 9, 19, 27, 32, 33, 39, 43, 50, 51, 52, 53, 56, 59, 66, 68, 70, 76, 80, 82, 84, 85, 90, 94 95, 98, 99, 102, 104, 108

I

Immunosuppressive drugs, 74, 101
Inspired air
  carbon dioxide, see $PICO_2$
  nitrogen, see PIN_2
  oxygen, see PIO_2
  concentration, 18, 19
Intensive care medicine, viii
  mechanical, viii
  pharmacological, viii
  supportive or replacement therapy, viii
Intermittent positive pressure breathing (IPPB), 55, 56, 78
Intracranial lesions, 29
Intubation, 61
Ionic balance, 35
Ischemia, myocardial, 76

K

Kidneys, vii, viii
Kyphoscoliosis, 107-108

L

Lactates, 48
Lactic acid, 27, 29, 39, 76, 87, 94
Laryngeal edema, 71
Lidocaine, 84
Liver failure, 39
Lungs, vii, viii, 15, 16
  damage, 41
  obstructive disease, chronic, see Obstructive lung disease, chronic

M

Magnesium, 35
Mechanical ventilation, 64-75
Microatelectasis, 67, 101
Minute ventilation, 16, 17, 28
Morphine, 80
Muscular dystrophy, 51
Myasthenia gravis, 98-100
Myocardial infarction, 29, 82, 84
Myocarditis, toxic, 100
Myocardium
  depression, 38, 39
  irritability, 86, 87

N

Nitrogen, 5, 6
  alveolar air, in, see PAN_2
  arterial blood, in, see paN_2
  capillary blood, in see $p\bar{c}N_2$
  inspired air, in, see PIN_2
  venous blood, mixed, in, see $p\bar{v}N_2$

O

Obstructive lung disease, chronic, 29, 33, 50-63
  compensated phase
    treatment, 55-59
  decompensated phase
    treatment, 59-63
Oxygen, vii, 5, 6, 7, 14, 15, 38, 45
  alveolar air, in, see PAO_2
  artetrial blood, in, see paO_2
  capacity, 9
  capillary blood, in, see $p\bar{c}O_2$
  content, 9
  hemoglobin-dissociation curve, 7-10
  inspired air, in see PIO_2

pressure, *see* PO_2
saturation, 9
solubility coefficient, 6
therapy, 43-44
toxicity, 43, 109
venous blood, mixed, in, *see* $P\bar{v}O_2$
Oxygenation, 15-16, 17-20, 22, 32-34, 68-69, 83, 84, 102, 103, 105
problems, 43-45

P

$PACO_2$ (CO_2 in alveolar air), 6
$PaCO_2$ (CO_2 in arterial blood), 6, 11
PAN_2 (nitrogen in alveolar air), 6
PaN_2 (nitrogen in arterial blood), 6
PAO_2 (oxygen in alveolar air), 6
PaO_2 (oxygen in arterial blood), 6, 7, 11, 102, 103
Papilledema, 38
Parenchyma, lung, 102, 108
  disease, 97, 99
  loss of, 52
$P\bar{c}CO_2$ (CO_2 in capillary blood), 6
$P\bar{c}N_2$ (nitrogen in capillary blood), 6
$P\bar{c}O_2$ (oxygen in capillary blood), 6, 7, 8, 14, 17, 20, 22, 23, 25, 28, 29, 31, 32, 34, 35, 36, 38, 45, 46, 48, 50, 52, 59, 67, 87, 90, 91, 92, 93, 95, 102, 105, 107
  arterial changes, 28-29, 40
  retention, 108
Peripheral nerves, 15
Permeable membrane, 3
pH, ix, 8, 11, 14, 15, 21, 22, 35, 38, 67, 76, 84, 85, 87, 90, 91, 92, 93, 94, 107
  arterial, 59
Phases, change of, 3-4
Phenformin intoxication, 29
Physiological dead space, 16, 17, 18, 28, 66, 101, 102
Pickwickian syndrome, 51
$PICO_2$ (CO_2 in inspired air), 6
PIN_2 (nitrogen in inspired air), 6
PIO_2 (oxygen in inspired air), 6
Plasma bicarbonate, 15, 16, 22, 23, 24, 25, 26, 27, 28, 29-32, 24-26, 45-49, 59, 67, 84, 92, 94. 95
  changes, 29-32
Pneumocystis carinii pneumonia, 101, 74

Pneumomediastinum, 62
Pneumonia, 19
Pneumothorax, 105
  tension, 70
  fulminating, 62
PO_2 (oxygen pressure), 7, 22, 33, 39, 52, 57, 58, 68, 87, 92, 107
  arterial, 32-34
  high, 42
  low *(see* Hypoxemia, arterial)
Poliomyelitis, 98
Positive end expiratory pressure (PEEP), 67, 102, 105, 109
Potassium, vi, viii, 35, 38, 40, 48
Potassium chloride, 48
Proteins, blood, 31
$P\bar{v}CO_2$ (CO_2 in blood venous blood), 6, 11
$P\bar{v}N_2$ (nitrogen in mixed venous blood), 6
$P\bar{v}O_2$ (oxygen in mixed veinous blood), 6, 11, 33, 34
Pulmonary edema, 19, 56
  acute, 27, 76-81
Pulmonary elasticity, loss of, 52
Pulmonary function tests, 51
Pulmonary infarction, 19

R

Radial artery, 20
Red blood cells, 7
Renal failure, 30, 39, 82
Respirator lung, 101
Respiratory abnormalities, 23
Respiratory distress syndrome, 19, 68, 101-105
Respiratory failure, 50
Respiratory insufficiency, 50
Respiratory muscles, 15
Respiratory rate, 16, 28
Rib fractures, 108

S

Sclerosis, amyotrophic lateral, 100
Septicemia, 76
SGOT, 39
SGPT, 39
Shock, 34, 91

hypovolemic, 82
lung 101
septic, 82
Sodium, 35, 41
Sodium bicarbonate (NaHCO$_3$), 12, 29, 35, 47, 79, 91
Solubility coefficient, oxygen, 6, 7
Status asthmaticus, 60, 62, 65, 82
Steroids, 58
Sympathomimetic drugs, 39, 83, 86

T

Tachycardia, 39, 70, 76
  paroxysmal atrial, 91, 93
Tetanus, 100
Tham, 48
Tidal volume, 16, 17, 18, 28, 44, 52, 65, 90
Tracheostomy, 44, 61, 96, 97, 99, 102, 104, 109

U

Ulnar artery, 20

V

Vascoconstriction, peripheral, 34
Vasodilation, central, 34, 38
Venous blood, mixed 7
  gas measurement norms, 11
  nitrogen, in, *see* $p\bar{v}N_2$
  oxygen, in *see* $p\bar{v}O_2$
Ventilation, 15, 22 45-49, 65-68, 83, 84
  alveolar, 17, 22, 25, 28, 40
  dead space, 17
  mechanical, 64-75
  minute, 16, 17, 28
  problems, 45-49
Ventilators, 64-65
Venturi masks, 44, 57, 59
Vomiting, protracted, 48

W

Wall nebulizers, 45
Waste products, vii
Water, viii
  gas solution, 5-7
  output, vii

RM161 .L36
Lapuerta / Blood gases in clinical practice